LIVING
WELL

WITH
MULTIPLE SCLEROSIS

A Comprehensive Travel Guide

THOMAS R. HOLTACKERS, PT (Ret)

ISBN: 978-1-54398-236-7 (print)
ISBN: 978-1-54398-237-4 (ebook)

CONTENTS

Prologue 1
About The Author 3

THE JOURNEY...5

My Journey Begins 5

Redirection 9

MULTIPLE SCLEROSIS AND LIVING WELL...13

Multiple Sclerosis: An Overview 13

Living Well: An Overview 16

A Summary 18

EMOTIONAL HEALTH...22

Emotional Adjustments to Multiple Sclerosis 22

Behaviors of Grief: The Victim Persona 26
   a. Break out of Your Emotional Shell 28
   b. Stop Living IN Your Story 30
   c. Avoid Apathy through Hope 33

Behaviors of Grief: The Survivor Persona 34
   a. Take Ownership of Your Multiple Sclerosis 36
   b. Let Go of the Past 37
   c. Begin Building on Your Successes 38

Behaviors of Grief: The Proactive Persona 39
   a. Find Strength in Your Weakness through Faith 41
   b. Seek Ways to Positively Re-Create Your Self 41

c. If You Are Not Creating Change, Change Will Create You 43

d. Experience the Stages of Change 43

Behaviors of Grief: The Advocate Persona 46

a. Turn Negative Circumstances into Positive Outcomes 47

b. Get Out of the Bleachers 50

COGNITIVE WELL-BEING...53

Concepts of Cognitive Well-Being 53

a. Improve Your MS Literacy 54

b. Become an Expert in Your Multiple Sclerosis 55

c. Be Proactive in Your Total Health Care 56

d. Prepare Now For Your Future With MS. 57

e. Exercise Your Brain 60

f. Optimize Your Cognitive Function 61

PHYSICAL FITNESS...65

Why Physical Fitness? 65

a. What You Do Not Use, You Lose 67

b. Prepare for the Future 69

c. Set Goals 70

d. Be Persistent: It Is Not the Day, It Is the Habit 70

e. Be Patient 72

f. Progress Relies on Positive Reinforcement and Delayed Gratification 73

g. Follow a Nutritionally Sound Diet 75

h. Follow Healthy Lifestyle Choices 76

i. Physical Fitness Feeds the Proactive and Advocate Personalities in You 77

The Building Blocks of Fitness 77
    a. What is Exercise? 78
    b. Bones 79
    c. Muscles 79
    d. Musculoskeletal Stress 80
    e. Effort Without Pain 82
    f. Fatigue 83
    g. Energy Management 87
    h. Endurance 91

Getting Started 94
    a. You Cannot Do It Alone 94
    b. Do Your Homework 95
    c. Get Ready to Start 97
    d. Where to Exercise 100
    e. Start Slowly–Take Baby Steps 101

Exercises 102
    a. Strengthening Exercises 102
    b. Strengthening Equipment 103
    c. Developing A Basic Strengthening Routine 105
    d. Variations of the Basic Routine 106
    e. Arm and Leg Strengthening Exercises 107
    f. Core Strengthening Exercises 107
    g. Flexibility Exercises 111
    h. Endurance Exercises 113
    1. Cardiopulmonary Endurance Exercises 114
    2. Muscular Endurance Exercises 116
    i. Other Exercises 116

**INTEGRATING SYMPTOM MANAGEMENT
WITH PHYSICAL FITNESS**...118

Symptom Management 118
    a. Muscle Weakness 120

b. Spasticity 120

c. Stiffness.. 122

d. Balance 122

f. Mobility.. 123

Bladder Dysfunction 126

a. Urinary System Function 126

b. Hydration 128

c. Bladder Management... 129

STAYING ON A LIVING WELL JOURNEY...133

Epilogue 135

PROLOGUE

Living with multiple sclerosis (MS) is a lifelong journey that requires you, the traveler, to make many adjustments to accommodate the rigors of life's winding road, filled with detours and potholes, while riding in a vehicle that is prone to breakdowns. The effects of life in general combined with living with a chronic, progressive disease upon this carriage you call your body are difficult and incomplete, for they not only affect the physical mechanical aspects of movement and power, but also the emotional quality of the ride. However, there is a way to endure these life changes, by following the living well with MS concepts. These concepts combine three essential parts—emotional health, cognitive well-being, and physical fitness—each acting as independent yet interactive components of the whole.

The path down which you travel in life in general may be plagued by hills and valleys, twists and turns; however, living with multiple sclerosis requires navigating the impediments of any number of possible symptoms, which makes your life's journey especially treacherous. *Living Well with Multiple Sclerosis: A Comprehensive Travel Guide* is a handbook for voyagers with MS who seek to better their lives through healthy living. It is not for sightseeing tourists, because adjusting to the harshness of multiple sclerosis is not a vacation.

This travel guide helps you make choices. You can choose to sit in a recliner or get up and move the best way possible. You can eat a candy bar or eat an apple; you can ignore the progression of the disease or take an active part in managing its symptoms. You can sit and cheer on others working for a cure, or you can get out of the bleachers and onto the playing field by volunteering and fundraising. These choices are up to all those who have the disease. What about you?

The concepts, principles, ideals, notions, techniques, and goals found in this travel guide can help you find options and make choices regarding wellness, health, and fitness, such as:

- becoming stronger, having more flexibility, and having more endurance, to maintain the best possible level of functional independence
- managing symptoms more effectively
- preparing for the recovery from a flare up of multiple sclerosis
- preparing for the ultimate victory: the cure and reversal of MS.

A one-size-fits-all approach to living well with MS would be as ambiguous as the disease. Therefore, throughout the text, terms like could, may, possible, some, approximately, might, many, and other nonspecific words are used to describe how wellness may play a role in managing your multiple sclerosis.

The concepts discussed in the following chapters are not intended to diagnose, prescribe, or treat the physical, mental, or emotional aspects of multiple sclerosis. Nor does the guide attempt to explain all the symptoms of MS that may affect you specifically. A qualified health care provider should be consulted before engaging in any exercise regimen, diet, over-the-counter medication, herbal supplement, fitness program, psychological counseling, treatment program, or any other implication of such expressed in the text of this book.

As you follow this travel guide toward fitness, you will realize that an explorer found the way ahead for you through the wilderness, plotted a course for others to follow, and retraced that path throughout life with the intention of expanding everyone's horizons. The author is that explorer.

ABOUT THE AUTHOR

Thomas R. Holtackers received his bachelor of arts in health, physical education, and recreation from Montclair State University in Upper Montclair, New Jersey, and a degree in physical therapy from the Mayo Clinic Physical Therapy Program in Rochester, Minnesota. He completed the coursework for professional development in the Counselor Education Program at Winona State College, Winona, Minnesota, and was a staff physical therapist at Rochester Mayo Clinic for over forty-two years. His work during those years included treating critically ill patients in intensive care units, patients with multiple sclerosis in the inpatient rehabilitation unit, and patients with upper extremity problems in the hand therapy department. He was the patient education specialist for the physical medicine and rehabilitation department in the section of patient education. He was a clinical and classroom instructor at the *Mayo School of Health Sciences* Physical Therapy Program. Tom is a former college athlete and high school health/physical education teacher and football coach. He has had multiple sclerosis for over forty-five years.

Tom was an active fundraiser for the Upper Midwest chapter of the National MS Society, having participated in local MS walks for over twenty-five years, and is a nine-year "sole survivor" of the 50 Mile Challenge Walk, which he completed in a hand-cycle.

He has been a volunteer with the National MS Society for over forty years, serving in various capacities at the national and chapter levels. His involvement includes teaching water and land exercise classes, facilitating self-help groups, training self-help group leaders, serving on chapter programs and medical advisory committees, and being a member of the Upper Midwest chapter's board of trustees. He has given many talks throughout the Upper Midwest states on physical fitness, sexuality, and management of MS symptoms including fatigue, spasticity, muscle weakness, and bladder dysfunction. He was a member of the National MS Society's National Programs Advisory Council, the Assisted Living Task Force, the Strategic Response Goal Steering and Implementation Teams, and the Midwest Regional Volunteer Leadership Council.

The author was also active in the American Physical Therapy Association on the state and national levels, the Mayo Clinic Physical Therapy Program Alumni Association, and the Rochester Center for Independent Living, and was a member of the Minnesota Governor's Council on Disability.

In addition to many MS Society local chapter awards, such as the Norman Cohen "Hope" Award, Tom was inducted into National Multiple Sclerosis Society's Volunteer Hall of Fame in 1999, was highly honored as the recipient of the National Multiple Sclerosis Society's 2010 National Volunteer of the Year, and was awarded a Lifetime Achievement Award for over thirty-five years of volunteering.

Tom was the recipient of the Corrine Ellingham Outstanding Physical Therapist Award from the Minnesota American Physical Therapy Association, and the Dale Schaffer Outstanding Alumnus Award from the Mayo Clinic Physical Therapy Program Alumni Association.

Tom presently resides in Mesa, Arizona, with his wife, Anne, and volunteers for the Arizona chapter of the National MS Society. He can be contacted at: mssux@mac.com.

THE JOURNEY

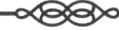

My Journey Begins

I started on my living well journey as a high school athlete and was guided along the way by the a principles of the athlete's attitude that embodies hard work, integrity, resilience, and discipline as the means to win games. For me, the ideals and concepts of fitness and sports competition being applied to coping with life have been strengthened through training and practice, playing high school and college football, and with my careers as a teacher, coach, and physical therapist. These principles were stressed by my parents, both of whom were athletes in their own rights, by my high school and college coaches, and by the instructors of the courses I took in college. I forwarded these same principles to the students in my classes and the young athletes I coached in football and track at the high school where I taught and eventually to the patients I treated as a physical therapist. Little did I know I would eventually apply these principles to my life's journey with multiple sclerosis.

When I decided to go into physical therapy, it was with the intention of teaching kids with disabilities these same principles. During my training, I was sidetracked from my original goal when I was exposed to the variety of situations that can be found in medicine. After I graduated from the Mayo Clinic Physical Therapy Program in 1972, I took a position at one of Mayo's hospitals treating critically ill patients in intensive care units. These patients were the sickest of the sick, yet despite all the equipment to which they were attached—ventilators and other various life support systems—I was still able to apply fitness principles to their care. Some did not survive their situation; however, there were many who did and benefited from my efforts.

During these early days of my physical therapy career I also started a journey with a career of a different type; I began having difficulties with the functioning of my central nervous system manifested through symptoms of severe fatigue, numbness, weakness, loss of balance, staggered walking, leg stiffness, and bladder problems that slowly progressed. I struggled to adapt to these problems without a diagnosis, though I had my suspicions. Finally, after seven years of frustration, anger, and doubt, it was confirmed: "You have MS." It was sort of a relief to hear those words for it finally provided answers for my symptoms. It also brought to the forefront a need to adjust to a life of physical decline, which was a very scary thought.

Despite the discouragement of some in the medical community with comments such as, "Go home and take it easy," "Don't fatigue yourself, for you may get worse," or "You can go on disability anytime you want," I chose to embrace the concepts of fitness and my life's philosophies, the principles of which were honed through training, trials, and battles on the playing field. I became engaged in many different venues of exercise with swimming, weight lifting, and wheelchair sports—basketball and road racing—all with the idea of trying to keep what I had not yet lost from the affects of the MS. I went against the conventional, ways of thinking for the time, which fortunately have been now discredited by most medical professionals. It is reassuring to know, with the growing medical research into the benefits of exercise and fitness for people with multiple sclerosis, that the new, twenty-first century philosophy supports my endeavors.

As a result of a gradual progression of my disease and a decline in my physical abilities, I had to change positions at work, which eventually proved to be to my emotional, mental, and physical advantage. I transferred to the rehabilitation unit, where I worked exclusively with patients with MS, which was one of my first applications channeling the negativity of MS toward a positive outcome for others and myself. Through treating my patients with MS, I learned a lot about the adaptations of exercise to a variety of MS symptoms and, because these adaptations not only applied to my patients but also to my own circumstance, I had begun the process of learning to become an expert in my own MS.

Unfortunately, because of the continued progression of my MS I developed a rapid onset of severe scoliosis that required fusion of most of my spine. After fourteen hours of surgery, three weeks in the hospital, three months of living in a body jacket, and a lot of physical therapy, I was able to go back to work. However, with the degradation of my functional abilities, I had to transfer, with much remorse, from the Rehabilitation Unit to a less physically taxing position in hand therapy. There I treated, from a wheelchair base, patients with injuries, surgeries, and conditions of the upper extremity of all types. Even though the circumstances of these patients were different from those I treated with MS, these patients also benefited from my fitness philosophies.

My career as a physical therapist at Mayo Clinic was managed through adaptation and accommodation on both of our parts. The Human Resources staff, along with my supervisors and physical therapy colleagues, were very supportive of my personal career goal of "retiring before have to go on disability." After 38 years, I achieved that goal! Even after retirement I continued to work part time in hand therapy before moving to Mesa, Arizona, with my new wife in 2014.

Early in my career as a person with MS, I began using my expertise as an athlete, coach, teacher, physical therapist, and person with multiple sclerosis to help others with MS. My first time volunteering in 1979 was conducting a water exercise program for people with MS at the local Recreation Center.

I recruited volunteers from the Physical Therapy School and others in the community to provide exercise for more than twenty people with multiple sclerosis. This was the start of a third career as a volunteer with the National MS Society. The Minnesota Chapter recognized the success of the program and soon I was being asked to volunteer in other activities. Conducting water- and land-based exercise programs at MS Camp, leading other exercise programs throughout the state, giving lectures regarding fatigue and exercise, along with MS Society committee participation soon filled my volunteer calendar.

During the years of constant readjustments to my disease, I was plagued multiple times with emotional unrest. Physical decline, the fear of financial demise, the emotional turmoil surrounding two divorces, and recovery from major spinal surgery was at the head of the list of circumstances toward this emotional unrest. I could not have coped with these changes without psychological help. I came to realize through intensive individual and group psychotherapy that was up to me to find the good in my situation. In one strange way, I became fascinated with the process my psychotherapists used to help me arrive at solutions to my problems. I began to use these same methods, only on a non-professional level, to help my physical therapy patients achieve their goals. My psychotherapy experiences also led me to facilitating MS Society support groups and, as my expertise in the small-group process grew, I eventually began to train group facilitators for the MS Society.

As my volunteer career progressed I also became involved with the American Physical Therapy Association, and was eventually recruited to lecture to physical therapists, nurses, and people with MS in other chapters throughout the country.

I have received many honors over the years for my efforts with the National MS Society and the American Physical Therapy Association, and they were very humbling; however, the greatest reward is knowing that I have been able to channel the negative aspects of my MS into something positive in helping others with MS while learning more about my MS than I could have ever learned in any textbook or at any lecture.

Redirection

The living well with multiple sclerosis philosophy became an essential travel guide in my life's journey. It has taken me a great while to change my life's direction as I encountered the rocky paths and canyons of coping with the future of a disease without cause and cure. Eventually this way of life with MS put me on the right course as I learned about the emotional, mental, and physical aspects of living with a progressive disease. Physical decline, divorces, surgery, and job changes provided many detours during my journey, but through the concepts of fitness, exercise, and competition that I began learning as a teenager, I was able to right my capsizing ship many times to get back on the right course.

One time in 2002 became a highlight and redirection of this journey for me. I had not taken care of myself very well prior to this aha moment. I had not practiced what I preached; I was just treading water and surviving the progression and life in general up to that point. Doubts about and fear of the future had crept into my consciousness. It was like the frog in the pot of slowly heating water; it was not to the boiling point, yet. I was out of shape and overweight. That year I got the flu. I developed a high fever and found myself stuck in my bathroom, overheated, and incapacitated, unable to move. Fortunately, I had just bought a cell phone and it was within my reach. I called 911 and, after an ambulance ride, I was admitted to the hospital dehydrated, weak, and very spastic. Intravenous fluids and antibiotics helped to stabilize my physical being, but my psyche had taken a major hit. It was a life-changing event. I had not taken care of myself as I had preached to my patients and clients with MS. I was admitted to the rehabilitation unit, which was also embarrassing, for it was the same department I had worked in previously. I was the patient now and not the provider, another hit to my psyche. My therapist, a former student of mine, hit me between the eyes with his approach to my therapy. It was tough, but positive and reassuring, the same traits I used with my patients. He got me on a comprehensive exercise program and followed through by going with me to the local athletic club to help me accommodate my fitness program to the available exercise machines. Intellectually I knew exactly what he was doing, but I humbled myself enough as to listen and learn from him. I was well on my way back to some level of fitness.

That experience was only the beginning of the new direction of my journey. Two months after my release from the rehabilitation unit, the Minnesota Chapter of the National MS Society announced a new fundraiser, the 50 Mile Challenge Walk to be held in September, only six months away. I was intrigued not only with the concept of the distance to be covered over three days, but also with the challenge of raising at least $1500 to enter the Walk. The problem was that I could not even walk 50 feet and I was not going to try to do it in my manual wheelchair, for the course was uneven, both up and down and side-to-side, which would destroy my forearm and shoulder muscles. I had heard of people using a hand cycle, which is a three-wheeled wheelchair with a bicycle rear wheel in the front that you propel by using a crank with handles connected to a sprocket with gears. I found and bought a used one and went out for a spin. After a mile, I thought my arms would fall off. However, I was not dismayed and vowed to raise the money and complete the Walk. I registered and started my training, which was slow and tedious. I was working fulltime, so I would get up at five in the morning two to three times a week to go out crankin,' then go home, shower, go to work, come home, and crash. Slowly, and I mean slowly, I gained strength and endurance. One of my greatest obstacles was the heat and my inability to sweat, which became a major threat to my well-being and a challenge for my fatigue-management skills. With each training session, I brought plenty of ice water and trained during the cooler times of the day. I trained all summer long and was able to work my training distance up over 20 miles several times. I knew I could do the 50 miles and I knew it would be hard, but that was the challenge.

I did it! I raised the money and completed the Walk; however, I had to take three days off from work. I was exhausted, but not dismayed; I signed up for the 2003 Challenge Walk. The following spring I began my training and fundraising, continued all summer long, finished the Walk and again had to take time off from work, but only two days this time. I signed up for the 2004 Walk and started a winter cross-training program at the athletic club with arm and leg strengthening and upper body exercise to maintain my arm muscle endurance. Again I trained all spring and summer, completed the Walk and, to my surprise, I did not have to take any time off work. I repeated my training schedule for the 2005 Walk and afterward I could have completed another one right then and there. In the process of training for four years, I lost weight, I felt stronger, and I had less fatigue and more energy that immensely improved my ability to complete my activities of daily living.

The 50 Mile Challenge Walk became a metaphor for my fitness, my fundraising, my life, and my destiny, to be as free as possible from the confines of multiple sclerosis.

In 2010, I completed my ninth 50-Mile Challenge Walk and I signed up for the tenth. However, I did not complete that Walk. Unfortunately, the Challenge Walk committee decided to change the dates of the Walk to try to capture a different segment of possible walkers. The previous Walks were in September, which is relatively cool for Minnesota, ideal for walking that far, at least for me. The new dates were at the end of June. The Minnesota summer was just getting started and the first day the weather was sunny and by nine in the morning it was ninety-five degrees with ninety-five percent humidity. I had only gone about five miles and had consumed all the ice water I had available when I had to stop. It was too dangerous for me to try to continue.

That same year I had major changes in my life. I met a wonderful, supportive woman. We got married and moved to Mesa, Arizona. I had intended to continue to use my hand cycle after we moved, but another powerful condition caught up to me. As I moved into the eighth decade of my life, the wear and tear of daily use of a manual wheelchair, wheelchair sports and recreation, and training for and completing nine Challenge Walks, the muscles of my shoulders began to become more prone to injury to a point of tearing several of my rotator cuff muscles. The injuries interfered with my activities of daily life, which eventually lead me to use an electrically powered wheel-chair that in turn required me to obtain a conversion van with a ramp and make modifications in our house.

All the changes that have caused a decline in my functional abilities were mostly a result of my progressive MS and aging, neither of which are under my control. Some of my decline was a result of my reducing the intensities of my exercise regimen because of pain and impaired function from the tearing of several shoulder muscles that were not repairable. Following the philosophy of living well with MS is my only recourse to acclimate to these new limitations

MULTIPLE SCLEROSIS AND LIVING WELL

Multiple Sclerosis: An Overview

Multiple sclerosis (MS) is recognized as an autoimmune disease, which simply means the body's immune system attacks itself. Normally our immune system fights off bacteria and viruses that enter the body. With MS, something triggers the body's defense to attack the cells that produce the insulation around the nerves of the brain and spinal cord known as the central nervous system. This insulation, called myelin, normally allows impulses to flow smoothly through the nerves that control the body's functions. In multiple sclerosis, the myelin around nerve fibers is broken down, causing the normal impulses to slow as they travel through the nerves—sort of a short circuiting, similar to what an electrical cord will do when the insulation is worn away. The condition is further complicated when the body heals the demyelinating injury, causing a hardening or scarring of the tissue around the nerve fiber. This process disturbs normal nerve functions, producing a variety of symptoms depending on what area of the central nervous system is affected, all of which may result in a variety of disabling situations. Multiple sclerosis may affect different parts of the central nervous system, so each person may have any combination of more than a dozen possible symptoms, each with a different level of involvement. These symptoms may include, but are not limited to, the following, which are not listed in degree of commonality:

- Fatigue—one of the most common symptoms
- Heat intolerance—fatigue worsens when body temperature increases
- Muscle weakness—may vary from muscle to muscle
- Spasticity—a resistance to muscle relaxation, causing stiffness in movement
- Bladder dysfunction—possible frequency, urgency, or incontinence
- Bowel problems—possible diarrhea or constipation
- Sexual difficulties—possible impotence in men; vaginal dryness and impaired genital sensation in women
- Numbness and tingling—may be of hands, feet, or other parts of the body
- Ataxia—a staggering gait
- Intention tremor—a shaking of arms, legs, or head with activity
- Visual impairments—possible double vision, blurriness, blindness, or others
- Pain—possible trigeminal neuralgia (pain in the face), spasms, lightning-like pain of the arms or legs, headache, or others
- Cognitive disorders—possible difficulty with memory, recall of information, word selection, or doing activities in an orderly fashion
- Depression—a result of the direct disease process (organic depression) as opposed to the indirect process caused by the reaction to the circumstances resulting from the disease process (situational depression)
- Dysarthria—difficulty with speech

- Dysphagia—difficulty swallowing

What causes the disease process to trigger is unknown and there is no cure or reversal of MS at this time. Most people with MS are diagnosed based on their symptoms and are usually in their mid-twenties and early thirties. There is a small percentage of people with MS who contract the disease before their teenage years and a small percent that are diagnosed after fifty years of age.

Some people who develop MS have an initial symptom referred to as a clinical isolated symptom (CIS) that lasts more than 24 hours. If they were to have another symptom after that initial symptom it would be considered to progress to MS.

Approximately eighty-five percent of people with MS have a relapsing-remitting form (RRMS) that is characterized by periods of disease flare-ups (relapses or exacerbations) followed by apparent calm (remissions). Approximately three fourths of people with relapsing-remitting MS are women. Similar to the unpredictability of a volcano, the intensities of the relapses of MS and the length of time between each event vary from person to person. Most people with this form of MS are treated with several immune system-modifying medications that have been shown to help reduce the intensity of relapses and increase the length of time of remissions. However, the long-term effects are yet to be fully realized. Unfortunately, not all people with this form of MS benefit from these medications.

At some point in time many people with relapsing-remitting MS stop having flare-ups and develop secondary-progressive MS (SPMS), which is more like the slow progression of a glacier. The length of time before this transition occurs varies from person to person, but a majority will make this conversion within approximately twenty-five years of getting the disease. Due to the relatively short history of using immune system-modifying medications with relapsing-remitting multiple sclerosis, it has not yet been determined if the rate and percentages of the conversions from this form of MS to second-ary-progressive MS will change.

Approximately fifteen percent of people with multiple sclerosis have primary-progressive MS (PPMS). This form has a glacier-like erosion of function similar to secondary-progressive MS. People with primary-progressive MS did not have clearly defined exacerbations and remissions like those with relapsing-remitting MS do. The rate and extent of erosion of abilities varies from person to person. There are several medications that have been used to try to halt the progression, but they seem to have only temporary benefit. Approximately fifty percent of people with primary progressive MS are men. A small percentage of people with primary progressive MS have a rare, rapidly progressive disease course formally called progressive-relapsing MS that causes extensive disability in a very short period of time, approximately five years. There are no medications to effectively halt or slow the progression of this form of multiple sclerosis.

In summary, multiple sclerosis is a chronic, progressive, demyelinating disease of the brain and spinal cord. There is no known cause, cure, or reversal of the disease process. The rate and degree of progression of the disease varies from person to person, as does the number and combination of symptoms experienced by each.

Living Well: An Overview

Living Well with Multiple Sclerosis incorporates the aspects of wellness while living with MS to help you develop emotional health, promote cognitive well-being, and become physically fit. These three parts of living well are intertwined and strengthen each other.

When you realize your own potential, are able to cope with the normal stresses of life, work productively and fruitfully, and are able to make a contribution to your community, you will have reached a state of great emotional or mental health. The positive dimension of emotional health is stressed in the World Health Organization's definition of health as contained in its constitution: "Health is a state of complete physical, mental and social well-being and not merely the absence of disease or infirmity."

Cognitive well-being involves gaining disease knowledge, also known as health literacy, which is defined by the U.S. Department of Health and Human Services as: "The degree to which individuals have the capacity to obtain, process, and understand basic health information and services needed to make appropriate health decisions."

Other components involve becoming an expert in your MS by learning the specifics of your symptoms and the latest treatment recommendations that might apply to their treatment, performing mind stimulating activities, and practicing cognitive-enhancing techniques.

Becoming physically fit is the process of preparing in healthy ways for a future condition or circumstance through appropriate diet, activity, and exercise that optimizes physical energy, strength and endurance, mental aptitude, and emotional fortitude. A report from the U.S. Department of Health and Human Services published in 2008, indicates the following:

> The health benefits of physical activity are seen in children and adolescents, young and middle-aged adults, older adults, women and men, people of different races and ethnicities, and people with disabilities and chronic conditions. The health benefits of physical activity are generally independent of body weight. Adults of all sizes and shapes gain health and fitness benefits by being habitually physically active. The benefits of physical activity

also outweigh the risk of injury and sudden heart attacks, two concerns that prevent many people from becoming physically active.

In 2008, reviewers from Denmark published an analysis of a large number of medical research studies on fitness and multiple sclerosis with the following conclusions:

> This review summarizes the existing knowledge regarding the effects of physical exercise in patients suffering from multiple sclerosis (MS). Furthermore, recommendations are given regarding exercise prescription for MS patients and for future study directions. Previously, MS patients were advised not to participate in physical exercise. During recent years, it has been increasingly acknowledged that exercise benefits MS patients. The requirement for exercise in MS patients is emphasized by their physiological profile, which probably reflects both the effects of the disease per se and the reversible effects of an inactive lifestyle.

Many smaller published studies have shown that exercise helps manage various symptoms such as spasticity, fatigue, weakness, bowel and bladder dysfunction, and even cognitive difficulties. Several studies have shown that people with MS who engage in fitness activities feel better about themselves, are more functional, and have a better-perceived quality of life.

A Summary

While the truth is difficult to face, it must be addressed; multiple sclerosis is a progressive disease, the future of which you may have done little to prepare for. While there is little you can do related to its progression other than receive the medical treatments that are presently available for you and recommended by your health care provider, you can have an influence in how you are able to adapt to the changes in your life that will occur as a result of the progression. How you weather this possible future has a lot to do with what you do in the present. This is where acquiring emotional health, cognitive well-being, and physical fitness come into play.

Unfortunately, old philosophies may have hindered development of the very concepts needed to compensate for the destructive nature of the disease. In the not-so-distant past, with the twentieth-century philosophy of managing multiple sclerosis, it was not unusual for some health care providers to suppress information regarding a person's MS. The reasons were partly out of ignorance and partly based on an unrealistic fear that patients would read too much into the specifics of the disease. This meant many with multiple sclerosis were left on their own to try to decipher rumor and speculation.

You may have been told that stress and excess fatigue would cause MS to progress, which you may have interpreted as, "Go home and rest." Unfortunately, inactivity causes loss of muscle strength, endurance, joint range of motion, and bone density along with increases in body weight, and, consequently, an increased risk of Type II diabetes, cardiovascular diseases, some cancers, and even depression. The combination of the progression of multiple sclerosis and aging can be compounded by unhealthy lifestyle choices of poor nutrition, smoking, and over-consumption of alcohol that will contribute over time to a decline in function, stealing the very core of life needed to deal with the disease.

Fortunately, a newer philosophy has emerged with twenty-first-century research encouraging appropriate activities directed at symptom management and maintaining function with anticipation of future disease progression. In other words, living well.

As you look at your present state of affairs and possible future related to multiple sclerosis, following the concepts of living well might be far from your mind. You might be saying to yourself, *How can I be live well and have MS at the same time?* This all takes time and energy and it seems like I'm fatigued all the time.

How you think of this concept may be influenced by what you have previously been taught or experienced. You may have discomfort caused by cognitive dissonance, which is a conflict between something new and something already thought to be right. This battle can cause guilt and anger because you may feel you have been making the right choices despite new, contrary evidence.

However, this bias may shed light on otherwise inappropriate behavior. MS not only erodes the body, it plays games with your mind and causes your spirit to bleed. You may mourn the loss of your past abilities while seeking comfort from emotional pain and physical fatigue. You might be insulating yourself in a cocoon of comfort that provides false security in the present for fear of a seemingly dismal future. You may seek relief from the discomfort of living with multiple sclerosis through destructive lifestyle behaviors because they feel or taste good. You may metaphorically sit in your rocker recliner, eat snacks, and watch TV all day long. Unfortunately, lack of exercise, poor nutrition, social isolation, and diminished mental stimuli add to the erosion of your body, mind, and spirit. Or, as the saying goes, *What you don't use, you lose.* This is especially true in respect to physical as well as mental abilities and emotional adjustments to the disease. Inactivity causes your muscles and bones to weaken, your heart and lungs to lose efficiency, and your metabolism to slow down—the latter of which promotes weight gain. These can cause you to lose self-esteem along with your overall effectiveness in life and how you view your masculinity or femininity, all of which are already being beaten up. When you add aging and other chronic diseases to this stew of strife, you are in trouble.

The primary purpose of the living well process is to help you optimize your overall function and ability to perform activities of daily living in a safe and appropriate manner.

This course of action is composed of the three individual yet interactive domains of living well: emotional health, cognitive well-being, and physical fitness. These spheres of influence will help you help reverse negative behaviors of neglect and ignorance. These domains of behavior exist individually and collectively for the success of the whole. Without one, the effectiveness of the others is less than optimal. The strength of living well is no greater than the weakest domain.

Having MS and living well may seem incompatible to you; however it is the very reason they must co- exist: multiple sclerosis breaks down; living well builds up.

The following chapters will explore the concepts by which the three domains of living well operate, briefly explain some of the more common symptoms of multiple sclerosis, and delve into their management through living well.

EMOTIONAL HEALTH

Whereas multiple sclerosis is a progressive disease, the rate and degree of which is unknown for each individual, your disease progresses differently from others with MS similar to the process of aging, both of which will cause change in your life. The changes of your body's function, processing skills, and emotional perceptions are exclusive to you because you are unique. How you adapt to the changes depends on all three domains of living well: emotional health, cognitive well-being, and physical fitness. While they are inter-related, you have powerful emotional forces acting upon the conscious and subconscious parts of your psyche, which means your emotional health will have the greatest influence toward the other two domains. Because of the progressive nature of multiple sclerosis, emotional health needs to be continually reinforced to retain a firm base; it is the process of coping with multiple sclerosis by redefining in positive, constructive ways, the self you see through your own mind's eye. When all three domains of living well work collectively against your negative reaction to the ravages of MS, you are better able to enjoy a more positive quality of life.

Emotional Adjustments to Multiple Sclerosis

The principles of emotional health relate to your reaction to multiple sclerosis that evolves through different levels of adjustment to grief, each assuming a personality of its own. These grief personalities co-exist and may come in and out of conscious focus because of several variables, the first of which is the progressive nature of the disease related to your emotional function. If you are having one exacerbation after another without a lot of time between, it becomes difficult to determine which personality you are exhibiting. The grief of loss is compounded with each attack, which means the phase of emotional adjustment of one attack is added to the emotions of each succeeding attack, stacking one grief process upon another. This is very difficult to manage alone, and it is for this reason that professional psychological help is highly recommended.

Another variable of adjustment is how you have dealt with emotional pain in the past. It could be more difficult to adjust to the ups and downs of MS if you have not coped in healthy ways with emotional upset prior to your multiple sclerosis diagnosis or the appearance of your MS symptoms. You may have resorted to coping with life's turmoil through use of drugs or abnormal behavior. You may not have developed a good support system such as family, friends, clergy, mental health care providers, and others to help you through the down times. This may be added to your emotional condition prior to MS. If you were dealing with some other emotional distress and then have to deal with MS, the grief is also compounded.

Your conscious recognition of the grief personality that is trying to influence you at the moment may also enter the picture. You may not be aware of which of these personalities you are exhibiting, for their expression can be very subtle. The more aware you are that they can be present, the better able you are to deal with them. However, this may be confusing because of your emotional maturation related to those personalities. The less mature personalities are more debilitating, but as you evolve the more mature personalities become a greater positive influence on your life.

Yet another variable in your adjustment to MS is your degree of motivation to nurture the positive personalities. Being aware of which personality is influencing your life at the moment and the enthusiasm with which you use the more positive ones will determine their effectiveness. This may also be influenced by your immediate situation of family, friends, neighbors, and work colleagues. The people around you are also grieving the losses associated with your MS and they, too, develop similar personalities in how they relate to you. How they treat you will have an effect on how you perceive the self you identify within your mind's eye: good, bad, or indifferent.

MS may not be the only stress with which you are dealing. Any adversity will produce an exhibit of one or more of these personalities. They all have influences on your psyche that help to mold your personality, the extent of which may be unknown.

As you evolve through these grief personalities you may advance to develop a higher level of emotional health only to regress to a former one when any of these variables influence your life. These fluctuations are normal, for while these personalities have succinct traits, they exist simultaneously, each vying for your attention. As the forward evolution of your emotional health increases despite the downward progression of your disease, the potential attentiveness of these personalities increases. With each new advance of the disease comes the potential for reversion to a less-mature personality. This is not to be feared because it is a part of the nature of loss and grief. However, when you acknowledge the process of mourning, it is easier to move forward again into a more mature personality like the ebb and flow of the tides of the oceans, a high and low among these identities competes for your attention. You might ask, *Which personality wins in this battle of dominance?* The answer is, *The one you feed*.

Unfortunately, feeding the lesser personalities takes an easier course through instant gratification and negative reinforcement of comforting behaviors, which usually occur with easing an uncomfortable feeling. Two examples of these negative behaviors are by eating low-nutrition comfort foods or avoiding the discomfort of fatigue by remaining inactive.

Feeding the positive personality is harder, but more reward-ing as it relies on delayed gratification such as being attentive to the foods that are beneficial to your health and the posi-tive reinforcement of being appropriately active and improv-ing your physical function. Building your emotional health on these latter two behaviors takes dedication and discipline, but provides a sturdier foundation upon which living well can be built.

Coordinating the concepts of emotional health with those of cognitive well-being and physical fitness helps to provide the appropriate emotional nutrients for a healthier, more mature personality, thus the better able you are to deal with the breakdowns and regression to a less-mature personality. This awareness of apparently losing ground increases with your emotional experiences, making you better able to develop breakthroughs toward an even higher level of emotional health. Therefore, while the breakdowns may seem to inhibit your upward development, following the concepts in deal-ing with each behavior will help you to make breakthroughs to higher levels with a positive overall result. The difficulty is being aware of the process and consciously trying to influence the change.

It is best to experience each personality at its own pace and time of progression so as not to have major relapses to a less-mature behavior later on. Without the proper order of the progression, the end result will be less than ideal, thus trying to rush the process and jumping to a more mature personality can cause you to regress more quickly to a less-mature behavior where you may get stuck. It would be like jumping from child-hood to adulthood without experiencing being a teenager. Without the experience gained in the teenage personalities, it will be more difficult to move on from the lower levels of your grieving reactions to MS, thus the progression to a higher level of grief maturity may take more time and effort, diminishing the overall result.

No matter the level or the order of progression to which you mature, you will still have breakdowns. The concepts of emotional health at each level will help you pull away from these breakdowns and help create more breakthroughs. You sometimes have to take one step back to gain two steps forward. Your recovery rate may vary with each episode, but relying on the training process of failure begets success moves you in a constructive, upward direction.

The most important philosophical belief you need to reiterate continually while working through breakdowns is, *Have faith in the process*. The processes succeed when you work them to your advantage. The process, which follows the concept of from weakness comes strength, is essential for progression. This is similar to the way you gain muscle strength with physical fitness, you have to fatigue your muscles for them to be stronger and more enduring. Therefore, with emotional health you may have to experience the pain of emotional upset to know how to deal with it, always keeping in mind you may need professional help to do so. No matter what the situation, you do have the potential of improving your emotional health by working through the evolution of grief personalities and redefining yourself in your mind's eye in ways that are more positive.

Behaviors of Grief: The Victim Persona

And since, in our passage through this world, painful circumstances occur more frequently than pleasing ones, and since our sense of evil is, I fear, more acute than our sense of good, we become the victims of our feelings, unless we can in some degree command them.

—Ann Radcliffe (1764-1823; English author)

You may feel like a victim of multiple sclerosis under the circumstances of having the disease through no fault of your own. This is a normal emotion; however, you are more of a victim of your reaction to having MS than having the disease itself. This sense of victimization grows by not dealing with your situation in healthy ways. If you internalize your feelings about what is happening, you may be projecting yourself into a worst-case scenario. This could be a result of having previous encounters with people with severe MS that may cause you to think, *That's what I am going to be like someday.* While it is not unusual to think you could be severely affected, it is very rare you will become that way. However, if you do not deal with your emotional turmoil surrounding these projections, you will become a victim of them. These perceptions may prevent you from participating in activities with others who have MS because you do not want to be reminded of how you could be in the future. That is why it is very important to remember that not all MS is the same; everyone progresses at a different rate and to a different degree of involvement.

If you are exhibiting the victim personality, you are most likely to exhibit the following emotions:

- Think MS is all about you.

- Grieve the past, deny the present, and fear the future.

- Live in a story about your past, all of which is a perception of the events surrounding your MS.

- Repeat often your story consciously and unconsciously; your story becomes your existence; it is like being stuck in your own *Groundhog Day* movie.

- Rely on instant gratification and negative reinforcement to avoid the pains of life.

- Have misdirected anger; anger at God for not sparing you, anger at health care providers for not having a cure or treatment, anger toward yourself and everyone around you, while exhibiting no anger toward your MS.

- Have unrealistic guilt of not trying to avoid the situation. *If only I had turned left on Main Street rather than turning right I would have*…. Feeling, *if only I had …* compounds any guilt over being in an unavoidable situation of having MS.
- Identify yourself as being MS, calling yourself an *MSer,* and blaming everything on MS.
- Be unaware of the need to change for the better.

If you can identify with some or all of these characteristics of the victim personality, fear not, for this is normal; it is another expression of loss and grief. However, it is best to avoid getting stuck in this behavior, which will keep you from evolving through the grieving process.

While there are many influences out of your control, you need to seek ways to work through how you react to the disease by being aware of the resources available to help you from your health care providers, the National MS Society, and other community resources, keeping in mind that you may need psychological help. However, you may eventually work through the victim personality maze by considering the following behavioral changes.

a. Break out of Your Emotional Shell

> ***Our negative experiences stick to us like Velcro ™, while our positive experiences slide right off us like Teflon™.***
>
> *–Rick Hanson Ph.D. (1952 to present; neuropsychologist, author)*

Multiple sclerosis is a progressive disease and living with it is a lifelong undertaking. In an attempt to accommodate the destructive aspect of MS, it is natural to try to avoid the emotional pain of change, but this avoidance may have far-reaching negative consequences. There is a tendency to avoid this pain by enveloping yourself in an emotionally protective shell, which comes about through the reinforcement of avoiding negative stimuli. That means it feels good to avoid the pain of the moment, but doing so adds to the need to avoid the pain. The sequence of emotional pain and then relief due to avoidance strengthens the avoidance. This cycling affect protects you by helping you to produce a cocoon of comfort and complacency to protect you from the pain, which only makes the pain worse the next time a major change occurs.

An example of the notion of comfort-seeking behaviors is the way you may have been avoiding fatigue, which is uncomfortable, debilitating, can cause injury and lessen social interaction. To diminish its effects there is a tendency to be less active, which provides only temporary respite. Too much inactivity in turn will make it more difficult to endure the activities that were fatiguing you in the first place, thus promoting more fatigue from the inactivity. The constant negative reinforcement of removing an unpleasant stimulus reinforces the idle envelope in which you are surrounding yourself. You find yourself in a vicious cycle of fatigue, inactivity, more fatigue, more inactivity, and so on.

Over time, unrealistic security becomes more entrenched in your lifestyle, which can affect your functional abilities. Enveloping yourself in a shell of emotional pain avoidance promotes a decline in self-worth, self-effectiveness, and quality of life. The effort to break free from these bonds takes knowledge, time, exertion, discipline, and persistence all of which makes the process therapeutic.

There are many examples in nature that use struggle to gain strength. The exertion to break out of its cocoon gives a butterfly the strength to fly and the same thing happens with a baby bird breaking out of its shell. Without the struggle, the butterfly and the bird may be too weak to fly.

Breaking out of your emotional shell and developing a healthier state of mind will help you endure the devastating effects of MS. While the support from family members, health care providers, and the National MS Society will help you succeed, only you can accomplish the potential progress you make.

To break out of your shell you need to develop the grit and guts of positively adapting to a negative situation. It takes work, discipline, and time for it is about your life with multiple sclerosis.

b. Stop Living IN Your Story

> ***I wake up every day, right here, right in Punxsutawney, and it's always February 2nd, and there's nothing I can do about it.***
>
> *–Phil (the main character in the movie Groundhog Day)*

All the talk of breaking out of your shell is encouraging, but the means to do so may sound vague. The process begins with trying to put your past in the past and putting your future in the present, creating possibilities for that future, and then beginning to act upon them in the present.

However, you cannot escape the influence of living with multiple sclerosis; it is part of you. You cannot change the past, but you can learn from it. A large part of your reaction to the past is how you interpret events of your life. Your interpretation of these occurrences is influenced by the impact they have on your life and is the basis of how you view the self in your mind's eye. These interpretations are a record of changes over time and may become the foundation of your existence. They become your story.

Telling your story becomes a very important part of coping with MS as it helps you verbalize emotions associated with the phases of grief. However, when you awaken each morning thinking about what you used to be able to do before MS and relive the events leading up to your loss, you are living in your story. You become like Phil in the movie, *Groundhog Day*, where he relives each day as the previous one and, also as in the movie, you continue to change your interpretation of what has happened. When you become stuck in your story and cannot continue to change the interpretation of what has happened, you become a victim of it.

There are several ways to get unstuck from this groundhog-day scenario of being a victim of living in your story.

- One is to tell your story to anyone who will listen—health care providers, family members, friends, clergy, or members of an MS self-help group—always keeping in mind that they may get tired of hearing it. Keep telling it repeatedly until you begin to find the good in it and, yes, there is good in your story, but you may need to search for it.

- Another way to get out of your story is to write it down on a piece of paper and then read it aloud to yourself with no one around. Continue to read it repeatedly until the story becomes pointless. This may take a while, but the intent of the exercise is to help you realize that, while you can learn from your past, living in your story is senseless because it holds you back from advancing with your emotional health. It is your interpretation of what happened to you, which often includes the embellishments of self-pity, unrealistic guilt, and misdirected anger, all of which are meaningless to your present situation. This will not help you prepare for the future. When you let go of your story, you will be better able to see how meaningful your life can be.

- Yet another way to help you let go of the past is to write a list of those aspects of your life that you lost because of your multiple sclerosis. List as many specific things whose loss you mourn as you can. They may be physical abilities, relationships, jobs, or finances; list anything that has caused you anguish. Take your time in compiling this list, put it aside for several days, then reread and then edit it. You may not realize your losses until you finish the list. This process may also dig up some old memories that you may have been suppressing because you have not dealt with them. When you are done with this list, literally place it in a nonflammable container and have a ceremonial burning of the story of your past. After you figuratively put the torch to your past, and begin to shed the protective shell of your story, you will need to concentrate on those positive aspects in your life and begin to prepare for your future. Your past is full of positive experiences that can give you strength, but your story about the negative events enveloping your multiple sclerosis has been holding you back from utilizing them. When you put your future in the present, you are better able to act upon those possibilities that you created and use them to reconstruct yourself in positive ways.

The process of developing a new foundation of emotional health begins with making a list of physical and mental tasks you are able to do under your present circumstances. Focus on the positive and tangible aspects of your life leaving nothing out, even the seemly insignificant aspects. Reinforce these positives in as many ways as possible, for they are how you diminish the negatives of your life.

As you begin to make changes in anticipation of the future, you will hopefully see that when you were stuck in your story you were living reactively, and when you direct your life forward you begin living your life proactively; you begin to break through the shell of victimization, stop living in a ground-hog-day scenario, and evolve toward the next personality, that of being a survivor. However, you may go in the opposite direction, thus developing an apathetic persona.

c. Avoid Apathy through Hope

> **We may have found a cure for most evils; but we have found no remedy for the worst of them all, the apathy of human being.**
>
> *—Helen Keller (1880–1968; American author, political activist, lecturer, first deaf and blind person to earn a Bachelor of Arts degree)*

Part of the upward progression from being a victim to a survivor and beyond is having and maintaining, hope. Anticipation of getting better and restoring a firmer hold on life generally comes with hope. Without it, the expectation of a positive view of the self within your psyche becomes more and more dim and the possibility of emotionally moving downward toward apathy becomes greater and greater. This may occur through having situational depression, which is part of the emotional grief process that may cause you to deteriorate into an apathetic personality and live indifferent to the world that is within your grasp. This will be devastating to you and those around you. Apathy may also occur if your evolution from the victim personality to the survivor personality breaks down. Apathy, because of lack of hope and giving up on life, can cause a downward spiral toward an abyss of total disregard for life. The apathetic personality may cause you to give up the battle either due to the disease process or your reaction to it. It is possible to move away from this dark place, but it takes a lot of time and effort with support from your family, health care providers, and mental-health professionals. However, only you can pull yourself up and away from this chasm, with hope acting as a strong component of the process.

Emotional health is a means by which you can avoid apathy due to your emotional reaction to your multiple sclerosis, and it can work to elevate your personality to a more productive one. However, keep in mind that if you have developed the apathetic personality and are moving forward again, you may exhibit victim personality behaviors again before moving on to being a survivor.

Behaviors of Grief: The Survivor Persona

Man's unique reward, however, is that while animals survive by adjusting themselves to their background, man survives by adjusting his background to himself.

–Ayn Rand (1905–1982; author, philosopher)

To make the leap from being a victim of your reaction to having multiple sclerosis to being a survivor is a gigantic step forward; however, it usually is a gradual transition over time. As you slowly begin developing a survivor personality you begin living your life to the best of your abilities, in spite of your MS. As you adapt to the physical and emotional changes, MS may hopefully become more of a hindrance or a nuisance rather than a restriction. Multiple sclerosis becomes a part of your life, but it does not control it except if you have a flare up. If this does occur, you may go back to a being a victim of your reaction to the new circumstances. You may then need to go through the process of working through your story again. Try not to be discouraged, because the concepts of breaking out of the victim mode from previous experiences will help you break through to being a survivor.

Hopefully, the more often this breakdown–breakthrough process occurs, the stronger you become and the easier it is to move forward. Like tempering steel through the process of heating and then cooling, the more often the process is repeated the stronger the product. You begin to realize that no matter what you do to prevent the disease from advancing, you may be able to get a stronger grasp of the perception that you will change and that you will have a healthier way of emotionally dealing with those changes.

If you are exhibiting the survivor personality, you are most likely to do the following:

- Focus on the here and now while still fearing the future.
- Be treading water; you are going neither forward nor backward with your reaction to the situation.
- Live your life in spite of the MS.
- May still refer to yourself as an MSer.
- Blame every inadequacy on MS: *I'm having an MS moment, that's why I forgot my keys.*
- Dismiss the anger and unrealistic guilt of having MS.
- Walk around the twelve-ton elephant sitting in the middle of the room called MS and not confront it.
- Hope for a cure and reversal of MS, but do nothing to help the cause.
- Be a cheerleader for others to volunteer and do fundraising.

- Contribute to someone doing the Walk or Bike Ride, but not participate yourself.
- Contemplate change, but take no initiative to do so.

If you can identify with some or all of these characteristics of the survivor personality, remember this is a normal process. However, you need to avoid getting stuck here, for the survivor personality is not really a healthy stopping point in life because you have the potential to evolve even further. You may need continued help from a mental health care provider and other resources available to you as well as engaging the following concepts.

a. Take Ownership of Your Multiple Sclerosis

There are two primary choices in life: to accept conditions as they exist, or accept the responsibility for changing them.

—Denis Waitley (1933-present; American motivational speaker and writer)

To deal with the enormity of living with multiple sclerosis and living a healthier lifestyle may seem overwhelming, but with the common, quiet courage we all possess within you can gain control over your reactions to the situations in your life over which you have control. As you awaken inner strengths, you are better able to struggle out of the emotional cocoon that is holding you back from living positively with a bad situation; you begin to be a survivor.

As you continue to stop living in your story and begin to be a survivor of your reaction to your MS, you will eventually need to take ownership of your multiple sclerosis in order to move through this personality. Taking ownership of anything places the responsibility of its future on the owner and in this case it is you; you own it, it is yours. For example, when you buy a new car you need to manage its upkeep. If you do not, you will pay the consequences of future problems that could have been avoided. Besides putting gas in it and keeping it clean, to help prevent a future breakdown you need to provide preventive maintenance such as changing the oil and getting a tune-up. These will help diminish the impact of any uncontrolled circumstances that may occur.

When you take ownership of your multiple sclerosis, you accept the responsibility for managing the parts of your life over which you have some control. A healthy lifestyle with proper nutrition and exercise, socialization, regular medical checkups for non-MS related issues, mental stimulation, and recreational activities might help prevent future problems. Yet, despite your efforts and not unlike your car, you may experience breakdowns that are no fault of your own. That is the reality of life, especially with MS. Nevertheless, to do nothing related to your maintenance in the present might make future health failures happen sooner and possibly to a greater degree, compounding the effects of multiple sclerosis in your life.

b. Let Go of the Past

If we open a quarrel between past and present, we shall find that we have lost the future.

—Sir Winston Churchill (1874–1965; Prime Minister of Great Britain during World War II)

Multiple sclerosis is a disease you developed through no fault of your own, though you may feel guilty for having it. You did not do anything to deserve your circumstances. You did not live in the wrong area, eat the wrong food, expose yourself to some toxic element as a child, or have a lack of something or too much of another.

If you have no control over your past, then why ponder events that you have no power to change? Face it, as the saying goes, *S**t happens*, and you accidentally stepped in a pile of it. You did not plan on acquiring MS. You did not say, *I think I'll get MS some day*. Of course not! It happened, and you need to break loose from the notion that it is your fault and you need to rid yourself of the unrealistic guilt you might have about your disease, for this may well be holding you back from addressing the future.

While you have little control over the progression of your multiple sclerosis other than the treatments that are available and recommended by your health care provider, you have some control over the management of your disease in the future. However, to begin to break through the negativity of unrealistic guilt about your past, you need to confront the control issues that may affect you in the present and will most likely influence your future. If your past is constantly being reviewed and re-lived in your present consciousness, it is difficult to prepare a future upon which to begin building in the present.

c. Begin Building on Your Successes

We climb to heaven most often on the ruins of our cherished plans, finding our failures were successes.

–Amos Bronson Alcott (1799-1888; American Educator)

You have experienced successes and failures in life; it is a normal process through which we learn. While you may feel having MS is a failure, there are many successes surrounding your reaction to the disease upon which you can build. They are there, but you have to look for them, as they may be hidden by your survivor personality. From an emotional health aspect, when you explore beliefs that can create possibilities for your future and then act upon them in the present, you will begin to evolve into a more positive personality. By learning from the negative experiences, you may be able to develop the perception of living your life positively with multiple sclerosis. Making the transformation from living in the past among your failures and preparing for the future through your successes is part of your emotional health journey. It is hoped this will lead you to the next level of adjustment by becoming proactive.

Behaviors of Grief: The Proactive Persona

Real freedom is creative, proactive, and will take me into new territories. I am not free if my freedom is predicated on reacting to my past.

—Kenny Loggins (1948 to present; American singer and songwriter)

Living your life as a survivor is an important response to MS, because it shows that you have moved beyond the victim stage where you were reacting to the disease with anger and guilt. And hopefully you have avoided apathy. However, this is not enough. There is more. A survivor does just that, survive, and you have been treading water alone in a sea of turmoil and the waters can get rough. As a survivor you were getting nowhere; you neither digressed nor progressed; you just existed in spite of your situation. It was a safe place to be, but not a productive one. You avoided the pain of progress, but it eventually caught up to you because you were not moving forward and upward.

At some point, you need to move beyond living life *in spite* of your MS by just surviving and begin to proactively transform your life in ways that reflect living your life positively *because* of your disease. In doing so you become a conqueror, not of your disease per se, but of your response to it. As you look at your situation, it is hoped that you realize the opportunities that are available to you. When you get to this point, you begin to be a victor over your reaction to your MS by responding. You start to channel the negative circumstances of your MS toward positive outcomes. You redirect the anger of having MS away from yourself and toward the multiple sclerosis.

The rate at which this process needs to evolve varies according to your circumstances. If you are having a flare up of your disease, you need to focus on recovery. If you are struggling with family or employment issues, concentrate on them. Do not deny the importance of the moment. As a person dealing with the changes brought on by MS and who has experienced evolving from the victim and survivor personalities, you have gained strength through adversity. You may even have reverted to a victim personality and then evolved forward into being a survivor, which made you stronger; however, to move into being a pro-activist when these issues resolve, you need to address the future as soon as possible. If you are exhibiting the proactive personality, you are most likely to be doing the following:

- Directing your anger toward your MS and away from God, yourself, and others.

- Fearing the future less and addressing it by creating possibilities for it.

- Starting to act upon those possibilities in the present.

- Becoming a participant, not just a cheerleader.

- Engaging in volunteering and fundraising activities as a team member.

- Beginning to re-identify yourself in positive ways related to your MS.

As you proactively address the twelve-ton elephant called multiple sclerosis that you have been avoiding as a survivor, you will begin to realize the good in your situation though you may have to look hard. Exploring the following concepts may help you make this transformation.

a. Find Strength in Your Weakness through Faith

That is why, for Christ's sake, I delight in weaknesses, in insults, in hardships, in persecutions, in difficulties. For when I am weak, then I am strong.

—2 Corinthians 12:10 (New International Version)
Apostle Paul (5-67 AD; Christian missionary)

Many people have risen above their adversity through faith, and a great example is the Apostle Paul, who was punished for it. Pain from torture during his imprisonment tormented him and he sought God's relief for which he received none and was told, *"My grace is sufficient for thee, for my strength is made perfect in weakness."* That prompted Paul to find strength in his own weakness.

You are experiencing a torment of your own living with MS and you have weakness in some form as a result. There are many opportunities to channel that weakness into something positive. Finding that pathway with a proactive personality is a part of your journey, but it cannot be travelled alone. Faith in a power larger and stronger than yourself will help you walk that path; seek that power and embrace it.

b. Seek Ways to Positively Re-Create Your Self

Life is not about finding yourself, life is about creating yourself.

–Anonymous

Multiple sclerosis changes your self-identity. It diminishes your self-worth, your view of your effectiveness in life and your sexuality or how you view yourself as a man or a woman. The extent of these changes depends on several factors, including:

- How you thought of yourself before your MS.
- The extent of your disease at the present.
- How you view your future.

As MS attempts to define the total you, you need to fight to maintain some level of feeling good in the here-and-now while grieving your departure from old identities. This grief often revolves around the loss of physical abilities and your perceptions of who you are. You grieve these through various phases of emotions such as denial, bargaining, anger, depression, shock, sorrow, and remorse. These phases may not come in any specific order and may even fluctuate.

While there is an end to the grief of one loss, the time it takes to go through the process varies. When you experience a new loss, you begin the grief process again, which when mixed with the unsettled grief of old losses can make living with multiple sclerosis overwhelming. You may develop a cumulative grief, which means the unresolved grief of one loss compounds the effect of the grief of other losses. Unresolved grief prevents you from moving forward and preparing for the future. All of these negative circumstances become stuck in your subconscious like Velcro™. They also become the basis of the story in which you became stuck and had become a victim.

To start the process of re-creating yourself, you need to acknowledge that you have a need to do so positively in order to counteract the negative identification you have created because of your multiple sclerosis. This takes time, effort, and realization of the need to change.

c. If You Are Not Creating Change, Change Will Create You

Change is the essence of life. Be willing to surrender what you are for what you could become.

—Anonymous

The result of your reaction to MS is to grieve your past, deny your present, and fear your future all at the same time. However, there is one certainty you cannot avoid; you will experience change. This frightening realization needs to be addressed, because it is an underlying reason to living well. Both MS and living well are future minded; one tears down, the other builds up. One you can do little about; the other, something about. In either case, adaptation to change is essential.

The principles of *Living Well with MS* will help you deal with the unpredictability of multiple sclerosis, but you need to change your present behaviors to anticipate change going forward due to those inevitabilities.

When you begin living your life in the future, you start moving from just surviving to being proactive. You start living your life because of your multiple sclerosis and start creating feasible possibilities that can be achieved for that future.

d. Experience the Stages of Change

You must be the change you want to see in the world.

—Mahatma Gandhi (1869–1948; leader of Indian independence movement)

Changes are most likely to occur because of your proactive personality as much as your proactive personality being a result of the change. However, to change present behaviors requires awareness of a need to change, a willingness to make changes, a plan to implement change, and means of reinforcing the change. This is often explained as the stages of change: pre-contemplation; contemplation; preparation; action and maintenance.

When you are in the pre-contemplation stage, you have no intention to change your sedentary behavior in the near future, possibly because you are unaware of the need to do so. This is most likely a part of the influence of the victim and survivor personalities. Moving out of this stage will most likely occur proactively, for it takes emotional motivation to begin the intellectual and evaluative processes. This stimulus may come from some inspirational encounter with a person, story, or motivational experience. Reading about other people's failures and successes with emotional and physical trauma is a good source of stimulus, and there are many to be found in bookstores, libraries, and on the Internet.

Contemplation is the stage in which you become more aware that a problem exists related to MS and your general well being. Raising your level of consciousness to be proactive in managing your multiple sclerosis begins during this stage, but you may not have made a commitment to start making these changes in your behavior. This trigger to change may come from an eye-opening experience through an encounter with another person with MS. One very effective way of becoming aware of the need to change is to expose your self to these types of experiences by being around other people with multiple sclerosis. You can join groups and clubs, attend educational meetings, and volunteer with the National MS Society and other MS organizations. These may go against your instincts as a survivor because you have been trying to walk around your problems with MS, but by working beside and with people with the disease, you will learn more about your MS than you may ever learn from a textbook.

Ultimately, the incentive to move forward has to come from within as you continue to build your emotional health foundation. This transition may take a while, but with time you develop a more conscious need to change with your increased awareness leading to preparation, the stage that blends your intention with new behavior. Your plan to start exercising and follow a healthier lifestyle is in the making, but you have not yet implemented it.

When you decide to begin to consider living proactively through living well, you start by countering old behaviors with new behaviors through substitution. Changing your dietary habits is a good example. Rather than having a candy bar for a treat, you choose to eat an apple. Both are sweet and satisfying, but the apple is more nutritionally sound. Another example would be having vegetables for a side to your main meal rather than pasta. Walking up one flight of stairs rather than taking an elevator or stretching your leg muscles rather than just sitting during television commercials are other examples related to your fitness.

The transition into the action stage of change requires the commitment of time and energy, but the results you see and feel will strengthen constructive behaviors through your proactive personality while reducing negative behaviors born during the victim and survivor persona development. This is especially true with exercise. Small advances in flexibility, strength, and endurance from appropriate exercise may be rewarded with the sense of small improvements in your ability to perform activities of daily living, which hopefully improves your perception of your quality of life. This reinforces the positive behavior, but do keep in mind that your level of function will vary from day to day because of the nature of multiple sclerosis. If you judge your level of functional abilities on just one day, you get a very narrow view. It would be like using the previews of coming attractions to judge the overall quality of a motion picture. Therefore, it is very important to look at these changes over time. It is also important to seek caring support from those around you, including family members, friends, or health care providers.

Maintenance is the stage of change in which you work to prevent relapsing into old behaviors while securing the gains achieved during the action stage. This stage usually begins some months after implementing your action plan and continues for an indefinite period of time. Reinforcement of positive outcomes overrides the continuing negative circumstances. Your MS does not go away, but you have a better grasp of its self-management.

The concept of creating positive change in your life helps motivate you to incorporate the other domains of living well, all of which strengthen your proactive re-creation. As you continue to grow in being proactive in your reaction to MS, you will hopefully start to seek ways of sharing your successes through volunteering and fundraising. If you were already active in these endeavors, you increase your involvement. You become more aware that you have been working toward the next level when you realize your negative behaviors and emotions can be channeled into positive outcomes by developing the advocate personality.

Behaviors of Grief: The Advocate Persona

It is a strange trade that of advocacy. Your intellect, your highest heavenly gift is hung up in the shop window like a loaded pistol for sale.

–Thomas Carlyle (1795–1881; Scottish satirical writer, essayist, historian, and teacher during the Victorian era)

To reach the point of being proactive with your reactions to multiple sclerosis you had to realize what you lost. This may have been painful for you to admit, but being realistic and honest about your situation helped you discard the shroud of sorrow you wore. There may be a sense of accomplishment over a seemingly overwhelming adversary producing an egotistic attitude toward life. Make no mistake, MS can be overpowering no matter what level you find yourself. The realization that multiple sclerosis is a progressive disease and needs to be stopped has to be brought to the forefront. With this realization and a commitment to raise funds for the research to stop MS progression, you have the potential to be a part of your own destiny: to be free of MS in your life. To help you with a new personal breakthrough you need to focus on what you have and how you can utilize your situation to create a positive change in your life and the life of others. For this to happen you have to become a participant in the cause; you become a crusader. But still you ask, *How do I do that, I have multiple sclerosis?* The following concepts will help you answer your own question.

a. Turn Negative Circumstances into Positive Outcomes

Build up your weaknesses until they become your strong points.

−Knute Rockne (1888-1931; famed University of Notre Dame football coach)

As previously discussed, your past is the past and there is nothing you can do to change it. Through emotional health you can utilize the experiences of the mistakes and successes of the past to nurture positive aspects of your present and your future. You do not completely forget the past because that is impossible and can be counterproductive. You do not turn off your negative past like a table lamp with a light switch, but you do try to lower the emotional barriers from the past similar to how you would lower the illumination of a dining room chandelier with a dimmer switch. The goal is to dim the destructive aspects of your past life and turn up those that are constructive in the present and future. Your past will always be a part of you and the emotions generated from the past can be very strong, but they can be channeled to produce positives changes in your life.

It takes time and energy to overcome your emotional reaction to multiple sclerosis' negative influence; however, through the living well processes you begin to make breakthroughs and start to make gains over your breakdowns. As you breach more barriers, you gain more confidence, which strengthens the belief in your ability to positively redefine yourself. This process is not easy and cannot be done alone; you may need professional help to assist you with confronting the very powerful emotions associated with living with MS. Mental-health professionals are not unlike other health care providers, they are there to help you deal with your problems. Ultimately, you are the one to follow the advice of those in whom you confide.

Anger is an example of one emotion that can be destructive or constructive depending on how you use it. Negative anger can trigger self-destructive behaviors, addictions, and other emotions such as depression. However, when anger is expressed in healthy ways the outcomes can be very positive by directing anger toward the multiple sclerosis and away from yourself, God, the health care system, and whatever or whomever you think is the root of its cause. As your misdirected anger is re-directed, the potential for positive change in your life and others is huge. When you concentrate your anger onto the very adversary that caused you to become angry, you begin to direct your life proactively toward the end goal of being free from MS for you and everyone else. That is the goal of the warrior advocate.

There are many examples of this process. Christopher Reeve, John Walsh, Lance Armstrong, and Candi Lightner have something in common. They all experienced negative, life-changing events. They all grieved their losses and most likely expressed anger over their situation. Yet they all were able to channel their grief to make a positive change in the world because of their situation.

- Superman actor Christopher Reeve fell from a horse resulting in quadriplegia and eventually started the Christopher and Dana Reeve Foundation for spinal cord injury research.

- John Walsh, whose son was kidnapped and murdered, started the *America's Most Wanted* television show to track down criminals throughout the country.

- After Lance Armstrong was diagnosed and treated for testicular cancer, he started the Lance Armstrong Foundation and used the sale of Live Strong rubber wrist bands to help fund cancer research.

- Candi Lightner founded MADD, Mothers Against Drunk Drivers, after a drunk driver killed her daughter.

It is very difficult to know how anyone would feel given similar circumstances, but the grieving process most likely included anger as one phase these people experienced. In each of the above examples, the achievements reached did not remove any loss. However, each person was able to channel anger and grief into something positive because of it. You may have the capability to do similar activities in your life, but you need to consider yourself a warrior and have some influence of change through your experiences.

b. Get Out of the Bleachers

> **Individual commitment is a group effort–this is what makes a team work, a company work, a society work, a civilization work.**
>
> *–Vince Lombardi (1913–1970; famed coach, Green Bay Packers of the National Football League)*

You want your situation with MS to change, but if you are not part of the process, you are not expressing an advocate personality. You may expect others to do the work while you sit in the bleachers and cheer for the players on the field. However, being a cheerleader does not make you a player. Never give up hope, but hope by itself is passive; it does not take effort to hope. It is when you get out the bleachers of hope and onto the playing field of volunteering and fundraising that you start to become an advocate. You become an active part of what you are hoping for and will feel good about yourself in the process. You become a member of a team of volunteers and fundraisers with the National MS Society staff, health care providers, scientists, researchers, and you. There is no I in team, but there is a U in volunteer and fundraising. When you become that U, you begin to be a part of the change you wish to see, ending MS in your life.

To begin the process of being a volunteer you first need to conduct an assessment of what you have to offer. List those attributes you possess that would be beneficial to the National MS Society and other MS organizations as a volunteer, which may include but are not limited to your:

- vocation, the kind of work experience you have
- avocational skills, hobbies and interests
- organizational skills
- physical abilities

- creative and innovative skills
- awareness of your present or anticipated needs
- financial resources.

When you use your positive attributes to further the mission of the MS Society, you become an agent of change in your life and the lives of others. Following this philosophy exemplifies a paraphrase of President John F Kennedy's famous words, "Ask not just what the National MS Society can do for you; ask what you can do for the National MS Society."

Volunteering and helping others with MS can help you cope with your situation. When you join the movement you will find there are many opportunities through the National MS Society to channel your negative circumstances into positive outcomes that will change you and others with MS. For example, you could do one or more of the following:

- Help mentor someone else with MS to work through their own roadblocks
- Facilitate a group or club.
- Volunteer at fundraising events.
- Offer to join a committee.
- Offer to fulfill one of the many other volunteer roles the National MS Society may have available for you.

Fundraising is the other part of exhibiting an advocacy personality. It takes money to provide the programs and research endeavors, much of which comes from fundraising activities in which you could directly participate or support someone else who is. Through your advocacy, you can inspire others to join you in fundraising, which will hasten the achievement of creating a world free from multiple sclerosis. With more people raising funds, the goal of curing and reversing the effects of multiple sclerosis on everyone will be that much closer and you will be an active part of that change and of your own destiny. Imagine how much closer we would be to this goal if everyone with MS were to be an advocate and raise money.

To be an effective advocate for the cause to end multiple sclerosis requires incorporation of your emotional health with the other domains of living well, cognitive well-being, and physical fitness. Following these principles is especially important, for it is the nature of the beast, multiple sclerosis, to cause you to have breakdowns. When disruptions happen, working a program of moving through the personalities of grief will help you deal with these dark days. This program involves identifying where you are in the process by stepping back from the emotional fishbowl in which you are swimming. Becoming mindful of the grief personality you are exhibiting will help you determine the point from which you start to evolve. This process starts by using the list of traits for each personality previously discussed as a guide, then work through the concepts of growth as best you are able.

COGNITIVE WELL-BEING

Whereas emotional health provides the foundation for your total living well journey, cognitive well-being provides the framework of knowledge and experience around which living well with MS can be constructed.

Concepts of Cognitive Well-Being

You can build your cognitive well-being infrastructure by educating yourself about multiple sclerosis in general and about your MS specifically. Following the philosophy that knowledge is power will better prepare you for the effects of multiple sclerosis on your life. One very powerful result of your investigation will be to realize that your MS is as specific to you as someone else's MS is to them. There are just more than a dozen symptoms that could develop through the MS disease process; each person has a different combination of symptoms anywhere from two to twelve or more, each with a different degree of involvement and rate of progression. The symptoms of your multiple sclerosis are unique to you and the more you know about how each might affect you and the treatments and management techniques that are available, the better able you are to cope with the disease.

As you become more aware of how your multiple sclerosis affects you, hopefully you will also be inclined to become more knowledgeable about other health care needs. The interrelationship between your MS and your general health becomes greater as you age, therefore the sooner you become aware of prevention strategies, the better your future will be. Learning is a lifelong endeavor in general and because multiple sclerosis is a progressive disease, cognitive well-being needs to be constantly reinforced and maintained based on the following concepts.

a. Improve Your MS Literacy

An investment in knowledge pays the best interest.

—Benjamin Franklin (1706-1790; author, political theorist, politician, scientist, inventor, civic activist, statesman, and diplomat)

The healthiest way to confront your multiple sclerosis is to learn as much about it as possible. Improving your understanding of MS in general and how it affects you specifically will expand your ability to manage it. There are many resources available to help enhance your health literacy regarding multiple sclerosis. To start your information gathering, try the following resources:

- Your health care provider.
- Patient education libraries of your local health care institution.
- The National MS Society and other MS organizations, which can provide written educational materials and recorded presentations by health care providers and people with MS.
- Reputable websites such as MayoClinic.com and webmd.com.

Rely on studies and reports published in reputable, peer reviewed medical/scientific journals that use a double blind format, which means the researchers and participants do not know who receives the real product or procedure and those who received a fake (placebo) product or procedure during the study. Avoid websites and literature that may be tainted with speculation and false information from unreliable sources promoting unproven, anecdotal claims of cures or use of herbal supplements, special diets, or procedures to treat multiple sclerosis. In addition, avoid claims of a product that you would need to buy. There have been many of these so-called cures, which have been proven false over the years. A few of them include, but are not limited to, the following:

- Drinking cow's colostrum (pregnant cow's milk).
- Removing metal fillings in the teeth.
- Using snake venom.
- Being stung by bees.
- Eating special diets (gluten free, vegetarian, or no red meat).
- Surgery on the arteries (carotids) in the neck to increase blood flow to the brain.
- Being exposed to hyperbaric oxygen (high-pressure air with high levels of oxygen).

Always check with your health care provider or the National MS Society if you are in doubt as to the authenticity of any claim or requests to enter a research project. There are always risks of doing anything out of the proven norm, both health and financially.

b. Become an Expert in Your Multiple Sclerosis

Try, try, try, and keep on trying is the rule that must be followed to become an expert in anything.

—W. Clement Stone (1902–2002; businessman, philanthropist, and self-help book author)

To work toward becoming an expert in your multiple sclerosis, try to know everything about the type of MS that you have, your symptoms, and which treatments are available to you. Always keep in mind that you will never reach that goal of knowing everything about your MS because it is constantly evolving, even if it is progressing very slowly. However, it is important to try. Your personal knowledge will help you increase your capacity to cope through your self-management program and help your health care provider be better able to assist you with your medical needs.

A good example of your need to know your MS is the phenomenon of having some of your symptoms, such as fatigue, spasticity, or poor coordination, differ in intensity from day to day for a variety of reasons. To deal more effectively with these fluctuations you need to look at individual symptom trends over time.

Remember, *Knowledge is Power*. Also remember that multiple sclerosis is progressive. You learning about changes associated with any new developments and how to cope with them is never ending. Like learning how to cope with multiple sclerosis, gaining knowledge is a life-long process.

c. Be Proactive in Your Total Health Care

Fundamentally, the answers to our challenges in healthcare relies in engaging and empowering the individual.

—Elizabeth Anne Holmes (1984-present; entrepreneur and founder and former CEO of Theranos)

While your focus is on multiple sclerosis, your knowledge about other aspects of your health is also very important. Regular checkups with your health care provider will help you avoid future problems where prevention is the key word and are unrelated to multiple sclerosis. Possible preventive measures may include but are not limited to:

- Cholesterol screening.
- For women: mammograms, self-administered breast exams, and pap smears.
- For men: prostate-specific antigen (PSA) screening and prostate exams.
- Colonoscopy.
- Blood pressure monitoring.
- Bone density scanning to check for osteoporosis.
- Skin lesion checks.
- Glaucoma screening.
- Vaccine updates.
- Periodic dental visits.

These are all dependent on the recommendations of your health care provider, who might have additional tests or procedures specific to your health needs. These might include monitoring heart disease, cancer, and other maladies through screening and preventive health. However, in the end, you need to be a self-advocate and the manager of your health because it is your body for which you are accountable.

d. Prepare Now For Your Future With MS.

I look to the future because that's where I am going to spend the rest of my life.

—George Burns (1896–1996; actor, comedian)

Your future with multiple sclerosis is unpredictable, as is the level of your physical and mental involvement from other causes, including the aging process. As you evolve through the emotional reactions to your disease through improving emotional health, you begin preparing for your future by joining the forces of emotional health with the concepts of cognitive well-being. Addressing life-planning concerns before they become an issue will help save heartache in the future. These life-planning concerns involve your financial, housing, and health care future, and also involve your personal relationships and the condition of your mind, body, and spirit.

Tips for preparing your future with multiple sclerosis may include, but are not limited to, the following:

- Become knowledgeable about the Americans with Disabilities Act that protects the rights of people with disabilities.

- If you work in a physically taxing job, consider changing vocations as soon as possible. Explore careers that permit movement within them to accommodate any future possible disability. Begin taking classes now and work toward a new degree or trade, if needed.

- If you are unemployed because of your multiple sclerosis, explore vocational rehabilitation agencies to help you get back into the workforce. The National MS Society may be able to help you with this process. There may be employment opportunities that could be managed from your home to accommodate future fatigue and decreased mobility issues.

- Consider accessible housing before you need it. Fatigue and weakness are common symptoms of multiple sclerosis that may be exaggerated with walking up and down the stairs of a multi-level home and put you at risk for injury. Though you may not need it now, consider moving into an all-one-level home with a floor plan that is without entryway steps and has an attached garage.

- Consider also moving into an accessible townhouse or condominium where lawn care and snow removal are taken care of.

- Explore your health insurance coverage and make changes now, if possible, to prevent future problems.

- Consider long-term care insurance to protect your assets. Be aware that you may not be eligible because of a pre-existing condition.

- Explore obtaining supplemental disability insurance if it is available to add to your employer's insurance to provide extra income if the need arises. Be aware that you may not be eligible because of a pre-existing condition.

- Become knowledgeable of any tax exemptions for which you may be eligible related to insurance, medical equipment purchases, and home modification.

- Reduce or eliminate your long-term debt as soon as possible to lessen the impact if your resources were to diminish.

- Try to maximize your retirement financial status through investment in Independent Retirement Accounts (IRAs). Seek a financial advisor to help you with this process.

Anything you do now that prepares you for a future of living with MS is an investment. It is similar to putting money in IRAs for when you retire, your cognitive well-being will gain interest over time.

e. Exercise Your Brain

> **I've got food and water and as long as I can exercise my mind and keep it nimble, then I'll be okay.**
>
> – Rob Walton (1945–present; eldest son of Sam Walton, founder of Wal-Mart)

Your brain needs to be exercised as well as your body. There is growing scientific evidence that performing regular, mentally stimulating activities will help keep the brain healthy and slow the onset of some age-related memory problems. Consider thought-stimulating activities such as:

- Maintaining social contacts with family and friends.
- Working crossword puzzles, Soduko, or word games.
- Playing cards and board games; there are many available on the Internet where you can play with people from all over the world.
- Reading books, newspapers, and magazines, many of which are available online, on electronic readers, or on CDs some of which may be available through your local library
- Listening to educational audiotapes CDs or watching DVDs or Blu-rays some of which may be available through your local library
- Exploring hobbies and taking community education courses.
- Enrolling in a course at your local community college or university; there are also many courses available through the Internet.

- Becoming active in your church, synagogue, or other religious or spiritual organization and in other community activities.

- Volunteering for the National MS Society, through which there may be opportunities available that permit you to volunteer from home.

- Volunteering at your grade or high school to help tutor students.

- Finding a part-time job.

There may be other activities in which you might be interested. Whatever the case, engage as much as possible in activities that stimulate your mind. Avoid mindless activities that do not offer learning, such as television programs and movies that are just entertaining. While these may be important to take your mind away from the stressors of your situation, too much of them are mind dulling and socially isolating, both of which are not what you need for optimum cognitive well-being.

f. Optimize Your Cognitive Function

I do believe that there are some universal cognitive tasks that are deep and profound– indeed, so deep and profound that it is worthwhile to understand them in order to design our displays in accord with those tasks.

—Edward Tufte (1942 to present; American statistician and professor emeritus of political science, statistics, and computer science at Yale University)

Cognition refers to mental processes that include attention, remembering, producing, and understanding language, solving problems, and making decisions. It is estimated that more than sixty percent of people with multiple sclerosis have some difficulty with these processes. If you are having difficulties in any of these areas it is best to seek professional help by contacting your health care provider. There are tests that can help you determine the areas of difficulty and level of involvement. There are also health care providers who can provide you with coping mechanisms to help you address these areas.

However, there are some ways you may adjust to these possible changes in your cognition.

- Attention—if you are having difficulties staying on task with a project or activity try these adaptations:
  - ◆ limit distractions of noise such as radios and visual diversions such as televisions
  - ◆ reduce other distractions such as uncomfortable temperatures or clothing
  - ◆ if you are distracted with a random thought, write it down so you can address it at a later time
  - ◆ organize and prioritize your tasks, then complete them in priority order pace yourself in completing the tasks so as not to be distracted by fatigue
  - ◆ if you feel you are being distracted, get up and move around for a minute or two, then settle back into the task
- Memory—if you are having difficulties remembering and recalling information, try these adaptations:
  - ◆ make lists of items or tasks: writing them down helps to them imprint into your conscious
  - ◆ repeat new names or items out loud; write them down
  - ◆ associate new or items with familiar references such as old images, words, songs/rhymes, or people; *Tall Paul, Mary Queen of Scots, or Michelle My Belle,* for example

- make up a silly short story around the items or tasks you want to remember. For example, if you were to make a grocery list try, I ate a ham and banana sandwich on wheat bread with a salad made of yogurt and peanut candy bars while applying deodorant after shampooing my hair.

- Executive Function Skills—if you have difficulty arranging and organizing more complex tasks such as planning a dinner party, going on vacation, or going to see your health care provider, try these adaptations:

  - use a calendar to write down an order of tasks needed to be accomplished leading up to the event

  - make a to-do list and then prioritize the list as to the order of completion of each task; keep it in an easily visible place such as on a bulletin board and cross out the tasks on the to-do-list as they are completed

  - keep labeled folders of forms and correspondence

  - keep all documents in one place such as a file cabinet that has a list of items in the file

  - keep bills in a box that is kept in a visible location

  - use auto pay to have bills automatically paid for

  - use electronic devices such as computers and smart phones to keep track of people and their addresses; have a back up system to secure their memory

  - designate certain days for certain tasks such as paying bills, doing the laundry, or cleaning the house; record them on your calendar as a reminder

- use alarms to remind you to start a task or make an appointment

Always keep in mind that as you experience more complex cognitive issues they need to be addressed by your health care provider to help you cope with this very frustrating symptom.

PHYSICAL FITNESS

Physical fitness is not only one of the most important keys to a healthy body, it is the basis of dynamic and creative intellectual activity.

—John F. Kennedy (1917-1963; thirty-fifth President of the United States)

Whereas the concept of living well is built on the foundation of emotional health and cognitive well-being is the infrastructure upon which living well is constructed, physical fitness is the power generated through appropriate exercise, fueled with healthy nutrition and supported through a positive lifestyle that drives the living well engine. Physical fitness is based on the following concepts that when followed may help you improve and maintain compliance with a lifelong program of appropriate exercise, symptom management, dietary habits, and healthy lifestyle changes.

Why Physical Fitness?

There are four major factors that may influence the possible loss of your strength, flexibility, and endurance and thus your functional abilities. The first two, multiple sclerosis and aging, are progressive processes in which the speed of onset, involvement, rate of decline, and ultimate degree of disability varies from person to person. The third process is inactivity, which may be promoted by symptoms of multiple sclerosis such as fatigue, weakness, depression, and spasticity and may cause the same functional decline as aging. Finally, poor lifestyle choices such as poor nutrition, smoking, and lack of regular medical checkups may lead to otherwise preventable health conditions.

While there is little control at this time over the progression of MS and the aging process, you do have some control over inactivity and poor lifestyle choices through the concepts of physical fitness. However, it is important to keep in mind that living well needs the interaction of all three components to help overcome the complexity of living with MS.

Your reaction to having multiple sclerosis may have influenced you to be less physically active. This could possibly be because you were told not to exercise, to conserve your energy, and to avoid fatigue. You may have difficulty moving fluidly because of spasticity, weakness, and poor balance. Your dietary preferences may have evolved into pleasure-seeking habits with poor nutritional value. The consequences of decreased physical activity influences weight gain, loss of muscle strength and endurance, decreased heart and lung function, and loss of bone density, all of which are preventable to some degree. In other words, you become overweight and out of shape. These circumstances, plus dealing with MS's overwhelming impact on your life, may discourage you from participating in physical fitness activities.

However, there is growing evidence from medical research that shows people with MS who exercise appropriately and routinely are able to:

- reduce fatigue
- increase strength
- manage spasticity and bladder dysfunction more effectively
- perform activities of daily living more safely and effectively

- feel an improvement in overall quality of life

- improve lung and heart function

- help prevent other diseases.

Weighing the positive impact of exercise and other aspects of fitness on living with MS against the negative aspects of multiple sclerosis by itself hopefully motivates you to engage in the concept of fitness. However, fitness is not an overnight success. The process of becoming more fit takes time, persistence, and a lot of support and effort. The results of your endeavors may be expressed through small improvements that may even go unnoticed in the beginning. Do not be discouraged, for eventually you will experience positive fruits of your labor that will grow and reinforce the whole process of living well with multiple sclerosis.

The following concepts will help you obtain your level of physical fitness.

a. What You Do Not Use, You Lose

Lack of activity breaks down the good condition of every human being, while movement and methodical physical exercise save it and preserve it.

–Plato (429–347 B.C.; classical Greek philosopher and mathematician)

You most likely have heard it before, what you do not use, you lose. You probably are not quoting that phrase in your mind when you are so fatigued that you cannot function effectively or safely without stopping and sitting down. However, keep in mind, your muscles, your teeth, and your friends have something in common; ignore them and they will go away.

As discussed in previous chapters, rest is a negative reinforcement of the behavior of sitting down to relieve a negative, fatigue. You may literally sit in your recliner, eat snacks, and watch TV all day long. Do that too often and for too long and you will lose strength, flexibility, and endurance. It takes the concepts of total fitness to undo the affects of inactivity by changing your attitude (emotional health) toward your symptom management by learning as much about the variables of fatigue (cognitive well-being), and finding exercises and other tools that promote its management (physical fitness).

The basis of physical fitness is engaging in exercises and healthy lifestyle choices that are appropriate for you to help improve overall ability to perform activities of daily living. Exercise will improve the ability to perform activities by:

- Strengthening parts of specific muscles not directly affected by multiple sclerosis and of those muscles not affected at all.
- Stretching muscles and joints to increase flexibility, help manage spasticity, and prevent tightness.
- Increasing endurance to help manage fatigue and appropriate body weight.
- Improving sitting, standing, and walking balance.
- Helping to prevent falls.
- Helping to prevent or reverse osteoporosis.
- Reducing emotional stress.
- Making healthy lifestyle choices to help prevent:
- Cardiovascular diseases.
- Certain cancers.
- Pulmonary diseases.
- Accidents and injuries.
- Following healthy nutritional guidelines to help:

- Maintain appropriate weight.

- Provide necessary energy.

- Maintain appropriate blood sugar levels.

- Prevent or reverse osteoporosis.

These are all achievable to some degree despite having multiple sclerosis, but it takes awareness and work, which are a part of living well with MS.

b. Prepare for the Future

The future starts today, not tomorrow.

—Saint John Paul II (1920-2005; leader of the Roman Catholic Church, first Pope from Poland)

If the cure and reversal of multiple sclerosis were to come about tomorrow, will you be physically prepared? Until that point, physical fitness will not reverse the damage from your disease, but it will help you prepare for that possible future. When that future begins to happen, it will take time and effort of exercise to regain gradually the potential function available for you and to start to undo the damage caused by your MS. When you the take time and effort now to undo the damage to your physical function as a result of your inactivity, you will spend less time and effort just preparing to endure the rigors of rehabilitation. Being in the best physical shape now will help restore overall function more quickly in the future. The training principles of discipline, persistence, and integrity that you develop now will also help you weather the aftereffects of an exacerbation.

c. Set Goals

> **When it is obvious that the goals cannot be reached, don't adjust the goals, adjust the action steps.**
>
> *— Confucius (551–479 BC;*
> *Chinese philosopher and politician)*

Setting goals and working toward them is an integral part of any fitness journey. While they can be classified as short term or long term, the overall goals of physical fitness are to:

- Improve and maintain your ability to perform your activities of daily living safely and efficiently.
- Help manage your symptoms of multiple sclerosis.
- Improve, maintain and coordinate your physical abilities with your emotional health and cognitive well-being.
- Improve and maintain your nutrition.
- Prevent complications due to poor lifestyle choices.

d. Be Persistent: It Is Not the Day, It Is the Habit

> **As long as we are persistent in our pursuit of our deepest destiny, we will continue to grow. We cannot choose the day or time when we will fully bloom. It happens in its own time.**
>
> *–Denis Waitley (1933–present; American*
> *motivational speaker and writer)*

Medical research continues to support the premise that fitness activities will help improve your ability to physically, cognitively, and emotionally manage your disease. For you to continue to pursue your fitness and functional goals requires confidence in the belief that what you are doing is beneficial and not detrimental. It takes time and persistence to continue your day-to-day efforts despite the ups and downs. As your multiple sclerosis moves forward, it tends to break down that confidence in the process. When you have breakdowns along your journey—and you will have breakdowns—use the concepts of emotional health and cognitive well-being to get back on the road toward your destination of living well with MS by making breakthroughs with your physical fitness.

The best outcome of your physical fitness regimen relies on a routine of exercise. However, it is not uncommon to do well on one day with one specific exercise and not with another. Then the next session, doing the same two exercises, the opposite may happen. One day you may only have enough energy to do a single exercise and on the next day enough to do five. There are several ways to address these variations:

- Maintain a habit of doing your exercises on scheduled days and time; do the best you can for that particular day.
- If you are having a bad day, remember that hopefully the next day will be better.
- Remember that exercise routines evolve over time.
- Try to maintain flexible expectations without procrastinating.
- Have a goal for the day but adapt according to the circumstances.
  - Consider that the daily variations of exercise outcomes could be affected by:
  - the variables of your symptoms, especially fatigue and spasticity.

- the time of day; morning may be a better time for you.
- your level of nutrition; when did you last eat?
- your level of hydration.
- your medications and time of day you take them.
- your activities prior to the exercise.
- your activities necessary after exercise.

When you have relapses in MS symptoms or in total fitness levels for any reason you may have reverted back to lower-functioning personalities. If that is the case, you will need to redevelop healthy habits to work toward breakthroughs and back to a higher functioning level. Whatever you do, do not give up because every day is the first day of the rest of your life and the opportunity to improve your life.

e. Be Patient

Patience is the support of weakness; impatience the ruin of strength.

– Charles Caleb Colton (1780-1832; English cleric, writer)

No matter the exercise outcome for that particular day, you can gradually improve if the potential for improvement over time is there. It is difficult to differentiate between what is lost from inactivity and what is lost from the direct effects of your MS and aging. Time and your health care providers will help you determine the difference as long as you continue exercising and you are patient with the results. It is also important to rely on how your functional abilities are affected over the long haul. It is hoped you will see an improvement in your ability to perform your activities of daily living, though it may take a long time. These improvements, as slight as they may be, are examples of delayed gratification and provide positive reinforcement of your program and your efforts.

However, at some point in time you will plateau with the results of your efforts. Do not stop doing the exercises. If you do, you will lose what you gained through all your hard work, and it will be at a rate faster than it took you to get to that point. Furthermore, the time to regain what you lost will take you longer than it took you to lose it. Do not forget that while you will most likely note fluctuations in your day-to-day functional abilities, believing in and allowing the fitness process to evolve will help you ride out these changes.

When you put the time, energy, and discipline into performing appropriate exercises specific to your situation, you will most likely note some improvement in one or all of the three major exercise domains of strength, flexibility, and endurance. While these advances may be small, they are positive results of your efforts, upon which you can build confidence. Use positive outcomes of your exercise program to reinforce the concept, and be patient.

f. Progress Relies on Positive Reinforcement and Delayed Gratification

Success is sweet and sweeter if long delayed
and gotten through many struggles
and defeats.

—Amos Bronson Alcott (1799-1888; American
teacher, writer, philosopher, and reformer)

Reinforcement of a behavior strengthens that behavior. Unfortunately, not all behavior is positive. As previously discussed, resting to avoid becoming fatigued reinforces the behavior of resting because it avoids an uncomfortable feeling.

Rest becomes a negative reinforcement of the feeling of relief of the fatigue. However, gaining strength and improving your performance of your activities of daily living is a positive reinforcement of the exercises.

Unfortunately, negative reinforcement is faster to employ and tends to be stronger because it feels good, while positive reinforcement takes longer and results are delayed. The slower onset of positive, feel good results are very powerful when they are recognized, but tend to be overridden with faster, negative reinforcement. You might say positive confirmation of your efforts is like Teflon™, it slides away very quickly, while the strength of negative reinforcement and instant gratification is like Velcro™, it sticks and hangs on for long periods of time.

It takes many positive results to counter one negative behavior. You need to hold on to and bank those positives and let them grow with interest to be successful. That is where the concepts of emotional and mental fitness play an important role in the support of your physical fitness. Positively seek ways to reinforce your efforts by documenting the results of your daily exercise regimen, which can help chart your progress. Always remember that daily ups and downs may seem that you are going backward, but be reminded that the positive results take time.

Set small, short-term goals and reward yourself in some small healthy way when you reach each and in larger ways when you reach long-term goals. Receive feedback from periodic follow-up visits with your physical therapist. There may be small advances that are sometimes hard to realize, so explore any improvement in overall function as feedback to your overall progress.

g. Follow a Nutritionally Sound Diet

And I believe that the best buy in public health today must be a combination of regular physical exercise and a healthy diet.

–Julie Bishop (1956 to present; former Australian Minister for Education, Science, and Training)

It is now well known by health care providers that a low fat, high fiber, balanced diet of fruits and vegetables, proteins found in dairy products, meats and fish, nuts and legumes, and whole grain foods along with appropriate routine exercise will help avoid potentially preventable conditions such as obesity, type 2 diabetes, cardiovascular diseases, lung diseases, and certain cancers whether you have MS or not. The practice of appropriate diet and exercise is recommended for everyone.

Supporting the energy required for healthy functioning and exercising of your body requires an appropriate fuel supply, which comes from ingesting the needed vitamins, minerals, proteins, fats, and carbohydrates of a nutritionally sound diet.

Diet has often been cited as a way to counteract (or cure) the effects of disease on the human body. While a nutritionally sound diet will generally provide the energy, vitamins, and minerals that are needed for life, fad diets and diets that rely on emotions instead of scientific research can do more harm that good. One factor that has been explored in the past is the subjective speculation that you should follow a diet of fish and gluten-free grains such as rice. This diet was based on the lower incidence of multiple sclerosis among certain populations of Asia whose diets consist of those foods, compared to a diet of red meat and gluten-containing grains such as wheat, which is the basic diet of many Europeans whose risk factors for MS are greater. Many years of medical research have proven that there is no known dietary practice that will prevent the onset or affect the outcome of your multiple sclerosis. Consult your health care provider and registered dietician or nutrition-ist for advice as to what diet is best for your situation.

h. Follow Healthy Lifestyle Choices

Follow your dreams, work hard, practice, and persevere. Make sure you eat a variety of foods, get plenty of exercise and maintain a healthy life.

—Sasha Cohen (1984 to present; U.S. figure skater, 2006 Olympic silver medalist, three-time World Championship medalist)

Exercise and following appropriate dietary habits are inte-gral parts of healthy living, however there are other lifestyle choices that you may have ignored. If you are a person with MS who smokes, consumes an excess of alcoholic beverages, and is unaware of the hereditary risk factors such as poor cholesterol levels, diabetes, cancer, and heart disease you are compromising your health. These will even make your life with MS more difficult to endure. While you cannot change your ancestry, you can reduce factors that promote those negative traits. Of all those possibilities, smoking is one very powerful influence. There is growing medical research that shows that smoking cigarettes is a forerunner to the onset of MS and if continued promotes the advancement of the disease process. The major message here is, "Stop smoking!" This is not an easy task, but you will benefit in the long run. Contact your health care provider for resources you may use to eliminate this health menace in your life.

Consult your health care provider for the specifics of your health risks. Knowing your other risk factors and acting to change behaviors that might support those negative factors is also very important. This concept of being an expert in your disease is a blending of the concepts of physical fitness and cognitive well-being.

i. Physical Fitness Feeds the Proactive and Advocate Personalities in You

> *Of the four personalities of victim, survivor, proactivity, and advocate that are constantly battling for your attention, which one wins? The one you feed.*
>
> *—Author*

It can be very difficult to remain an advocate for the cure and reversal of multiple sclerosis because MS has many effects upon which the others feed. When your MS worsens and life becomes more difficult, the victim and survivor traits kick in. These are normal reactions that need to be witnessed and acknowledged but not maintained, or you will lose what you gained from your efforts prior to the event. When you recognize the regression to those more primitive, just hanging on behaviors, you will once again need to restart the progression of feeding the proactive persona and then the advocate persona through the living well process. Getting started with something positive is the first step, followed by increased efforts. As you continue to grow in confidence, strength, and endurance those positive results, though delayed, are nourishment for living well with MS.

The Building Blocks of Fitness

If you take minutes a day to take care of your mouth, the odds are you'll take the next steps needed to take care of your whole body, like exercising and eating healthy. It's a building block for other healthy habits.

— Gretchen Bleiler (1981 to present; American former professional skateboarder)

a. What is Exercise?

True enjoyment comes from activity of the mind and exercise of the body; the two are ever united.

— Wilhelm von Humboldt (1767-1835; Russian philosopher)

Exercise is the basis of physical fitness and involves a large array of possible activities that are also used to address very common symptoms of MS. These activities may include, but are not limited to, the following:

- improving strength, flexibility, and endurance
- increasing balance and coordination
- promoting relaxation
- addressing specific multiple sclerosis symptoms such as fatigue and spasticity.

To address the principles of exercise is important to have a working knowledge and better understanding of how the body responds to exercise. The specific, scientific aspects of exercise can be found in many physiology texts and other resources, however, consider the following to gain a basic knowledge of your body related to exercise.

b. Bones

There are 206 bones that make up your skeleton. They play an important role in the function of the body. Specifically they:

- Protect vital organs such as your brain within the skull and your heart and lungs within the ribcage.
- Provide attachments for your muscles to produce joint motion, thus being able to perform physical activities.
- Serve as a reservoir of calcium and other minerals.
- Provide a source for your blood cells.
- Other functions such as the bones in your inner ear.

c. Muscles

Muscles act upon the bones that make up the joints of your skeletal system to provide movement. They are attached to the bones with tendons, which are somewhat elastic and not to be confused with ligaments, which have very little elasticity and connect bone to bone. When the impulses from your brain stimulate your muscle cells, a percentage of those muscle cells contract or shorten, pulling on the tendons to produce movement at the joint. Resistance to the movement causes more muscle cells to be engaged to produce the same motion. This relationship between the numbers of muscle cells firing verses the amount of resistance provided to the muscle is closely regulated by the nervous system. It normally triggers just the muscle function necessary to overcome the resistance. This prevents you from using fifty pounds of force to overcome five pounds of resistance, which would be very inefficient. The more resistance, the more muscle cells are activated; the less the resistance, the fewer muscle cells are needed. If there is too much resistance for the muscles to overcome, there will be no movement. Most muscles have some activity most of the time even though you are not moving. This activity is called tone, which acts to support the body against gravity and to maintain a readiness of the body to act in time of need.

Most muscles are grouped into one of two main categories: those that bend joints and those that straighten them; they oppose each other. For example, when the quadriceps muscles located on the front of your thigh are activated to contract and shorten to straighten your knee, the hamstring muscles, which normally bend your knee and are located on the back of the upper leg, have to relax to allow their lengthening for the knee to straighten. In reverse, when you bend your knee, your hamstring muscles contract and shorten and the quadriceps muscles relax and lengthen. Under normal circumstances, such as with walking and running, this is a smooth, efficient, and rhythmic motion.

There are other muscles that slide, glide, or rotate joints; they all have opposing muscles that function in a similar way as with the bending/straightening of joints to produce a coordinated motion. Other muscles play an important role in holding your body up against the pull of gravity. These postural muscles may not produce movement, but must work to maintain your posture and hold you stable by preventing unnecessary movements.

d. Musculoskeletal Stress

Producing stress is the foundation of maintaining and strengthening your bones and muscles. Appropriate amounts of stress over time result in an increase in strength, whereas not enough of this stress causes bones and muscles to weaken.

Too much stress over a short period of time damages them. Muscle cells grow in size and strength when they are broken down from the stress of resistance and then given several days rest to rebuild. The process is slow, thus the cycle of stress and rest has to be repeated over a long period of time for the best results.

When muscles are not given enough stress they will weaken. The longer the muscles go without stress, the weaker they become. Other than the direct results of MS and aging, inactivity is the greatest contributor to the process.

Your bones will remain strong with appropriate amounts of stress, which comes from frequent weight-bearing activities such as walking, and when your muscles are used for activities of daily living and with resistance exercises. Your bones will weaken over a long period of time (decades) without enough stress. As they slowly deteriorate, they lose their mineral density producing osteopenia and eventually osteoporosis. Severe osteoporosis may result in mini-fractures of the spine simply from gravity and poor posture. Severe osteoporosis may also cause any of your bones to break if you fall. You are at a greater risk of developing osteoporosis if you:

- are a woman—there is an increased risk following menopause
- smoke
- drink large amounts of alcohol
- are inactive for long periods of time
- have a diet poor in essential minerals and vitamins.
- get older

Overall, musculoskeletal stress is an important component of muscle and bone health when appropriate amounts of force are applied to your body. Too much or too little will compromise your muscle strength and bone integrity.

e. Effort Without Pain

Another essential component of exercise is effort; however, you may have been taught that effort equals pain. The old adage *No pain, no gain* is very misleading. Pain is a result of damage and is a message to back off the intensity and frequency of the exercise, or to stop exercise altogether. If an exercise causes an ouch during its performance, it probably means you are doing harm. This type of pain from exercising can be a result of very small tears in the tendons that are attached to the muscle. If these rips in the tissue do not heal, continued trauma can lead to tendonitis (inflammation of the tendon), complete tearing, or even detachment of the tendon from the bone.

An over-stretching or tearing of ligaments that help hold joints together or even from small fractures in the bone, especially if they are osteoporotic, can also cause pain. Therefore, ouch pain is bad and needs to be addressed before resuming exercises that caused the pain. If the damage is minimal, it may go away after several days of rest, ice packs, and over-the-counter pain medication following the manufacturer's instructions. If you are able, it is preferable to take a non-steroidal anti-inflammatory drug (NSAID) such as ibuprofen or naproxen, but never take two or more NSAIDs at the same time. To help prevent upsetting your stomach, take an NSAID during a meal. Consult your health care provider if the pain does not go away or returns after resuming the exercise, even with less intensity. Your health care provider needs to be informed before starting any new medication, even over-the-counter drugs.

Another type of pain, caused by microscopic tears in the muscle tissue, is referred to as delayed onset of muscle soreness (DOMS). This pain usually occurs several hours after completing resistance exercise and may last for several days. It is generally not felt at rest, but is present when the muscle is used. Refining the type and intensity of your resistance exercises and gently stretching your muscles after exercise may help to prevent this type of pain.

There is a good pain, which is the mild soreness you may experience after starting a new exercise or increasing intensity of one you have been doing. This type of discomfort generally means the by-products of muscle metabolism have not yet been removed from the tissues through increased blood flow, which takes more time when you are just starting a new exercise.

Overall, a good rule to follow is, *If it aches today from what you did yesterday, you did too much yesterday.* Therefore, it would be best to back down on the intensity of the exercise that caused the pain and advance more slowly the next time you perform that specific exercise. Also, gently stretch the muscle that is sore prior to resuming the exercise, use an ice pack, and take an over-the-counter pain medication that you would normally use for a headache, preferably an NSAID if possible. If the soreness does not lessen and go away in a day or two, or if you have difficulty differentiating pain from fatigue or stress, contact your health care provider for assistance. In addition, make sure you are doing the exercise correctly. Contact your physical therapist if you need assistance with learning how to do your exercises.

f. Fatigue

The success of your physical fitness program is dependent upon your understanding of how your multiple sclerosis relates to the various components of living well. One of the greatest aids to your success in this matter is the power of knowledge. This is particularly relevant to fatigue and management of your energy expenditure.

Fatigue is the most common symptom of multiple sclerosis and is basically a result of the loss of myelin or the insulation that is wrapped around the nerves within your brain and spinal cord. This demyelination causes slowing or blocking of nerve function, which could affect you physically, mentally, and emotionally. The amount of involvement in each of these domains varies greatly from person to person. Overall, fatigue could be caused by any combination of the following, which are directly related to your multiple sclerosis:

- poor nerve conduction
- muscle weakness
- spasticity
- so-called MS fatigue or idiopathic lassitude that suddenly occurs without a specific cause
- depression
- heat intolerance.

Most people with MS experience heat-related fatigue. This is due to increases in core body temperature, which is the temperature inside your body and not the same as your skin temperature. As your core body temperature goes up, the functional ability of a nerve fiber affected by MS decreases. This results in exaggerated symptoms and is often referred to as the Uthoff phenomenon, named after a German physician of the late 1800s, Dr. Wilhelm Uthoff. He observed that when his patients with multiple sclerosis who had optic neuritis became overheated, their eyesight worsened, but when they cooled down their eyesight went back to previous levels. Until modern diagnostic techniques were developed, patients who were suspected of having MS could be given the hot bathtub test in which they were immersed in hot water for a period of time. If their symptoms worsened and then improved after cooling, they were given a diagnosis of multiple sclerosis.

There are many possible causes of increased core body temperature. Some of these causes may have a greater influence on your fatigue than other causes. It is important to take all of them into consideration. Some possible causes and means of managing them include:

- We all experience a diurnal (twice daily) temperature change where core body temperature is normally lower in the morning and higher in the evening. The amount of fluctuation varies from person to person, but it could be up to a degree centigrade. Consider doing the more strenuous activities of daily living in the morning.

- The temperature and humidity of the room or outside air will influence core body temperature. Consider air conditioning to help manage the temperature and humidity of your exercise environment.

- You absorb heat being in the direct sun. Consider staying in the shade and avoiding the sun during the middle of the day when the sun's rays are more direct.

- Hot foods and drinks such as soup and coffee will briefly help increase core body temperature. Consider consuming cooler foods and drinks on hot days.

- The process of digesting food generates heat. This is known as the thermogenesis of digestion. Some foods create more heat than others do through this process. Consider what kinds of food you eat, when you eat them, and the activities you plan to do afterward.

- Large muscle activity produces heat, which means the more physically active you are the more heat that is produced. Consider doing more strenuous tasks that involve your large leg muscles in the earlier hours of the day.

- Some people with multiple sclerosis are unable to sweat, which normally is the body's way to reduce surface heat through evaporation. Check with your health care provider if you think you have difficulty sweating.

- Other considerations of managing heat intolerance may include but are not limited to the following:

    ♦ if you are unable to sweat, wear light, loose-fitting cotton fabrics that breathe

    ♦ if you perspire, wear fabrics that draw or wick perspiration away from your skin

    ♦ layer the clothes you wear to accommodate changes in your environment

    ♦ wear as little as possible under the circumstances, environmentally as well as socially and aesthetically

    ♦ consider cooling from the outside-in with cooling vests, collars, hats, and towels

    ♦ consider cooling from the inside-out by drinking ice cold liquids. Keep in mind that using ice cold liquids is not ideal for replacement hydration due to excess sweating.

There are other variables, which are indirectly related to your MS that may have daily influences on your fatigue over which you have some control. These may include but are not limited to:

- not being active enough
- being overweight and out of shape
- smoking

- poor nutrition
- increases in core body temperature
- depression
- lack of sleep
- not drinking enough liquids
- practicing poor energy management.

Identifying any of these in your life provides you with the opportunity to develop possibilities to gain control over their management, which will help you with your activities of daily living, meeting your total fitness goals, and improving your quality of life.

g. Energy Management

Whereas fatigue is a lack of energy, the main concept of energy management is to avoid overwhelming fatigue through the efficient use of your daily energy allowance. Like other aspects of living with multiple sclerosis, your energy may vary from day to day. A good analogy is that you receive a certain amount of money you can spend on any given day, but any balance left over from today cannot be saved for tomorrow, which means you cannot conserve your energy. You do not always get the same amount from day to day; one day you may have one hundred dollars worth of energy to spend, the next day you have seventy-five dollars worth and the following day you may have ninety dollars worth. There is no way to predict how much energy you will have until you attempt to spend it. If you spend more energy dollars than you have for a given day, you go into energy debt. Like any other debt, it has to be paid off and in this case it is through rest. This debt could possibly carry over into the next day before it is paid off. In other words, if you are fatigued today from what you did yesterday, you did too much yesterday.

Part of energy management is learning from hindsight, developing conclusions of what caused you to expend too much energy for that given day and avoiding it the next time. Ideally, you try to spend what you have today without having a balance or a debt at the end of the day. Learning how to manage your energy expenditure takes time and attentiveness to the variables over which you do have some control and weathering the unpredictable variables over which you have no control.

The basic energy management concept is to practice, activity, rest; activity, rest; activity, rest, and so on. This notion may be applied to each task and activity you plan for the day. The idea is for you to use some of the energy you have available for a period of time during a specific activity and then rest. The amount of activity and the length of rest vary with your level of energy at that point in time and with how fast you use that energy. If you use too much energy for any one activity and do not rest, you may not have enough energy for other activities. There are other tips you can use to help manage your energy:

- List your activities for the day and prioritize the order in which you want to complete them; try to do the hardest first, the second hardest next, and so on.

- Keep in mind that you may not be able to accomplish all of your scheduled activities in a given day because your energy allowance may be less than expected (you are having a fifty dollar day instead of a one hundred dollar day).

- Be flexible with your expectations so if you run out of energy you can put off that activity to another day.

- Avoid procrastination. It will only make your energy spending less efficient.

- Slow down. How fast you use your energy is very important. If you try to speed up your activity to get it finished before you run out of energy, the quality of the task diminishes and you become less efficient. It is like speeding up to get to the next gas station before your car runs out of gas. The car's miles per gallon go down as you speed up, so you run out of gas sooner.

- Pace yourself. Use your energy at your tempo. Communicate with family members and co-workers as to what your energy levels are when you are interacting with them. Go at your pace rather than theirs.

- Stop to rest at the first feeling of diminished energy. However, make sure you do not rest too long, just enough to get re-energized.

- It will take experimentation to get the feel of how much is too much and how much is too little of rest and activity.

- As always, keep in mind that every day is different and you should expect the unexpected.

- Avoid the tendency to feel unrealistic guilt for resting even though you may not look tired while others around you who do not have MS continue to be active.

- Maintain open lines of communication with family members, co-workers, and friends about the amount energy you feel you have that specific day and time. Their expectations may differ from yours, but you have to go at your pace as opposed to theirs. Trying to keep up with them when you do not have the energy may promote resentment, anger, frustration, and depression for all who are involved.

- Plan ahead to allow for more time to complete tasks and break up each task into segments. Tackle the hardest part of the task first, go at a steady pace, and take periodic rests. After you are done, relax for a while before tackling the next task.

- Use adapted equipment to help complete tasks more effectively, efficiently, and safely, such as:
  - canes and crutches for balance and weakness
  - splints, braces, and orthotics for weakness and paralysis
  - wheelchairs for long distances
  - other aids for activities of daily living, such as bathing equipment and dressing aids
  - check with your health care provider for the appropriate devices for your situation.

Lack of activity causes your body to lose strength, flexibility, and endurance, all of which lead to less energy. While exercise will cause short-term loss of energy, pursuing physical fitness over time may help improve your overall amount of energy.

There are other considerations to energy management. Talk to your health care provider if you are experiencing any of the following:

- Urinary frequency and urgency causing you to go to the bathroom many times a day.
- Autonomic nervous system dysfunction, causing a poor heart rate and blood pressure response to increases in activity, which has been identified in some people with multiple sclerosis.
- Emotional distress, especially depression.
- Spasticity and stiff movement increases energy expenditure.
- Balance problems may increase energy expenditure; consider using a cane or walker for stability.

- Walking long distances may be very fatiguing; consider using a wheelchair for those occasions.

- Interrupted and lack of sleep caused by:
    - depression
    - urinary frequency
    - restless legs or periodic limb-movement disorders
    - sleep apnea syndrome, which could be caused by an obstruction of your windpipe often characterized by loud snoring during sleep and sleepiness during the day.

There are some prescription medications and over-the-counter supplements such as caffeine that are used to try to increase energy, but they may have unwanted side effects. Always check with your health care provider if you want to explore their use.

h. Endurance

Endurance is the ability to perform an action repeatedly. For instance, your capacity to perform a function such as walking involves:

- A power source provided by your muscles.

- A cycle of fuel delivery and waste removal provided by your blood vessels, heart, and lungs, referred to as your cardiopulmonary system. This cycle involves:
    - your blood, laden with nutrients picked up through the digestive system, is pumped by your heart into your lungs where it picks up oxygen from the air you are breathing in.

- your heart then pumps this blood from your lungs through your arteries, delivering its nutrient cargo to your muscle cells where they use it as fuel for muscle function.

- the work of your muscle cells to produce carbon dioxide and other waste products that are picked up by the blood that deposited the oxygen and nutrients. This mixture is transported through your veins to your lungs where they are exchanged for more oxygen to start the whole cycle over again.

- removal of some of the chemical byproducts of cellular metabolism by cycling the blood through other organs such as the liver and kidneys.

As your muscles become more active, they need more oxygen thus producing more carbon dioxide and other waste products. This results in a greater need for the delivery and removal cycle, causing your breathing and heart rate to go up accordingly.

Your overall endurance is largely dependent on the efficiency of cycling oxygen and nutrients to your muscles and removal of carbon dioxide and chemical waste byproducts. While the primary drive of this cycle is through the normal actions of your heart and lungs, there are several other reasons why may you lose this endurance:

- Your muscles are weakened because of your MS.

- Your diet is of poor quality, reducing the supply of necessary nutrients for the muscles and causing you to gain weight.

- Your cardiopulmonary fuel delivery and waste removal system is faulty, a result of poor-quality blood vessels from lack of exercise, poor nutrition, and buildup of cholesterol.

- The nicotine in tobacco is causing your blood vessels to get smaller.
- Smoking, which produces carbon monoxide. Carbon monoxide takes up space in the blood that is meant for oxygen.
- Poor exchange of oxygen, carbon dioxide, and waste products at the muscle cell and in the lungs and other organs.
- You are too inactive, causing your:
  - fatigue to worsen, resulting in more inactivity thus producing a cycle of fatigue, rest, more fatigue.
  - skeletal muscles to weaken, reducing their effectiveness with transferring oxygen into the muscles and removal of carbon dioxide and waste products out of their cells.
  - respiratory muscles to weaken, reducing your lungs' ability to pump air in and out.
  - heart to reduce its ability to pump blood.
  - weight to increase because you are burning fewer calories.

There is a slight possibility that there is a malfunction in your heart's ability to increase rate and pressure due to an abnormal autonomic nervous system response that is found in some people with MS. This part of your overall nervous system helps your body to function automatically, affecting such things as hair and nail growth, blood pressure, heart rate, blood vessel size, and perspiration. A loss of your ability to sweat indicates an abnormal autonomic nervous system response and may be life threatening in high temperature environments. If you suspect you are sweating less than previously, consult with your health care provider.

Getting Started

So what do we do? Anything. Something. So long as we just do not sit there. If we screw it up, start over. Try something else. If we wait until we have satisfied all the uncertainties, it may be too late.

—Lee Iacocca (1924–2019; American businessman)

a. You Cannot Do It Alone

A person who treats himself has a fool for a patient.

— (paraphrase of an old medical axiom)

There are many resources from which you may draw support for your physical fitness endeavors that may include, but are not limited to, the following:

- To get started in a physical fitness program, begin by seeking input from a physical therapist as to what specific exercises to do that address your physical limitations.

- Speak to other health care providers as to any possible health risk factors that may be affected by exercise.

- Explore ways to adapt your daily living activities to incorporate physical fitness into your daily lifestyle.

- Multiple sclerosis is a family affair, so also include your family in your plans and speak to them about the possible changes in the priorities of daily life that would affect them.

- Explore community resources that will support your efforts, which include but may not be limited to:
    - National MS Society and other MS organization programs
    - the YMCA
    - private health clubs
    - community education classes
    - community swimming pools.

These resources are designed to help reinforce and add to the program your physical therapist developed for you, but not to replace it. Ultimately, you may have to do some of the exercises everyday and at home with the support of those resources.

b. Do Your Homework

Before taking that first step in your fitness journey, begin with a plan that will make your journey become more feasible. To help with these matters, consider exploring the following:

- Contact your health care provider prior to starting any new exercise program, especially if you have no experience with exercise. This is very important for your safety and well-being, as there may be aspects of your MS or other health care issues that might prevent or restrict you from doing one or more exercises safely. This is especially true if you have:
    - heart disease or risk factors such as high cholesterol, or a family history of these risk factors.

- high blood pressure, diabetes, arthritis, or asthma or other lung diseases.
- osteoporosis or a history of recently broken bones, especially those of the spine.
- a recent history of smoking.
- had a joint replacement.
- an uncertainty about your health.

- If exercise was a part of your pre-MS life you may have to modify your approach to getting started because your symptoms may interfere with your attempts to exercise at previous intensities, leading to unexpected consequences.

- Check with your physical therapist about the most important exercises to start with to meet your specific needs, especially if you are not sure of which exercises to do. Your therapist could also help guide you to more general fitness goals.

- Develop short-term goals based on improving specific functional abilities and managing your symptoms.

- Set long-term goals based on improving overall fitness, preparing for a recovery from a relapse of your disease, and diminishing long-term health risks.

- Develop an athlete's attitude toward fitness that relates to your life in general. This mentality, which includes practicing and playing hard, seeing failure as an opportunity to succeed, and working toward a goal with discipline and hard work will help you compete against your foe, MS. A good understanding of these concepts can be found in various books by successful sports coaches such as:

- John Wooden (basketball), who co-ed a book titled *Coach Wooden's Pyramid of Success: Building Blocks for a Better Life*
- Joe Gibbs (football), who co-authored a book titled *Game Plan for Life*.

c. Get Ready to Start

There are many situations that need to be addressed as you get ready to start exercising so consider other logistics involved with your plan. Pick a time of day that fits into your present schedule keeping in mind how the energy expenditure effects of exercise may affect the rest of your day. If possible, find someone with whom to work out, preferably someone of similar abilities, such as a family member or friend. Always keep in mind the old adage about the best-laid plans. There will be breakdowns that, it is hoped, lead to a breakthrough. Planning ahead and referring back to the concepts of emotional and mental fitness will help you weather these ups and downs.

As you prepare for and implement your exercise program, keep the following recommendations in mind while taking notice they are the same as with performing your activities of daily living:

- Be safe:
    - keep the area of exercise clear of obstructions.
    - have a chair available to sit and rest if needed.
    - do not rush; perform the exercises under control.
    - ask for help when needed.
    - plan to rest between each exercise if needed.
    - plan to rest after the exercise period before you go on with your day's other activities.
- Maintain the quality of each exercise:

- explore how to manage your energy before, during, and after exercise.
- follow the concepts of core body temperature management.
- exercise in a cool environment—air conditioning, fans, out of direct sunlight.
- wear cool, layered clothing to be gradually removed as your temperature rises.
- wear cotton if you cannot sweat.
- wear moisture wicking clothing if you sweat a lot.
- consider wearing a cooling vest.
- keep hydrated; remember that dehydration increases weakness, spasticity, and fatigue
- if you cannot sweat, drink cool or ice water to help lower your core body temperature.
- if you sweat a lot, drink water and liquids with electrolytes (sports drinks) that are closer to room temperature to permit better absorption in your digestive system.
- exercise in the earlier part of the day when your body temperature is generally lowest.
- do not exercise right after a meal, your core body temperature rises with digestion.

- Prioritize your time and energy. Everything else determines the when, what, and how much.
- Take your time as you progress through the exercises each day.
- Follow the concept of activity-rest, activity-rest, activity-rest between exercises.

- When doing a specific exercise, adapt the concept of activity-rest for your repetitions by using repetition-pause, repetitions pause, repetition pause.

- Increase the pause between repetitions as you experience more fatigue and less quality of the repetitions.

- Stay in control while performing the exercise; do not rush.

- Use proper body mechanics and posture. For example, use your leg muscles rather than back muscles when lifting objects.

- Breathe properly when doing an exercise. Exhale with the effort of the exercise. Do not hold your breath.

- Take periodic rests before engaging in more vigorous exercises.

- Stop when you get too fatigued.

- Balance your workout week with strength, flexibility, and endurance exercises.

- Determine your level of effort by what the exercise feels like rather than the amount.

- If you experience pain, stop; when the pain subsides start again with less effort

- Do not try to push through the pain

- If you experience pain that does not go away with a specific exercise, stop doing that exercise and try a different one that does not cause pain.

Keep in mind the quality of the exercises needs to be emphasized first and then the quantity. Following the adage of practice makes perfect is misleading because if you practice something in the wrong way, then you will become perfect at doing it wrong. Rather, think practice makes permanent and practice doing the exercises the correct way.

d. Where to Exercise

While there are many exercises that can be done at home, exercising around other people provides social interaction, which may assist you in staying motivated and consistent. However, with exercises that require equipment, where you exercise depends on several factors, which may include but are not limited to:

- your financial resources
- transportations needs
- equipment needs
- community resources.

Each exercise site has its own mixture of equipment. Try to find the best and most convenient place for you. Explore your neighboring YMCA, school and recreation center gymnasiums/pools, as well as private health and athletic clubs. For specific exercise programs, investigate resources such as the National MS Society, community education, and senior center programs.

There are exercises that can be done practically anywhere such as push-ups, sit-ups, stretching, elastic band, or isometric strengthening exercises and many others. You can use plastic shopping bags filled with various sized water bottles to create hand-held weights. Change the amount of water to increase or decrease the resistance. Brisk walking, if you are able, or even wheelchair dancing can be aerobic.

The most important where is wherever you are able to do something. It beats the alternative of doing nothing.

e. Start Slowly—Take Baby Steps

The best way to start your fitness journey is to choose a day and time that best fits into your daily/weekly schedule. Do a minimal number of exercises with one to two sets of eight to ten repetitions until you get comfortable with the quality and quantity of the routine and until you understand how the exercise session affected your symptoms and activities of daily living. Try to start with a balance of strengthening, flexibility, and endurance exercises, keeping in mind the benefits of each, which may be in response to your specific symptom management needs. For example:

- Monitor your progress by documenting your efforts in a notebook or on a computer spreadsheet.
- Add to your exercise regimen slowly as you accomplish initial short-term goals and add new ones.
- As you become more fit, slowly add more exercises over time to meet your long-term goals.
- Reassess your short- and long-term goals from time to time to accommodate changes in your function.

Start by doing stretching exercises, followed by strengthening, and ending with endurance for up to approximately 15 minutes each, once or twice a week. After several weeks of trying to maintain a consistent routine and assessing how the exercises affect your energy levels afterward, gradually add and subtract exercises depending on the level of benefit from each. Try to keep the number of days a week you exercise the same. After another several weeks of doing an expanded routine of exercise, add to the number of times a week you exercise.

As your workouts get longer, you might consider dedicating every other day for strengthening and different days for endurance. In addition, try to keep stretching each day you workout. Warm up before strengthening and endurance exercises and cool down with endurance exercises; this will help to prevent injury. Make small changes as you feel improvement and continue to adjust the exercises depending on how they affect your symptoms. Always keep in mind the daily fluctuations of living with your multiple sclerosis and practice your energy management skills.

Exercises

All parts of the body which have a function if used in moderation and exercised in labors in which each is accustomed, become thereby healthy, well developed, and age more slowly, but if unused they become liable to disease, defective in growth, and age quickly.

—Hippocrates (460–370 BC; ancient Greek physician)

a. Strengthening Exercises

To strengthen muscles, they need to face enough resistance to cause some level of muscular fatigue. The intensity and degree of this overload is dependent on the muscle's overall condition and the level at which you can safely endure. When muscles are resisted to a point of intense fatigue, a feeling is produced that is often referred to as a burn, which is due to a buildup of chemicals in the muscle cells. Typically, this feeling should not be misinterpreted as pain unless the burn does not go away after a minute or two or if it is repeated even with light resistance. If the burn persists, this may indicate an overuse and injury of the muscle, which needs to be addressed before repeating the exercise.

You do not need to produce a burn for your muscles to get stronger, however it is one indication of maximum effort. A good way to measure fatigue of the muscle without a burn is to provide enough resistance and repetition to begin to diminish the quality movement of the joint on the last few repetitions of the exercise. This means the effective repetitions are the last one or two of the final set that you can just barely do with good quality, which is considered to be an acceptable level of effort. If you are unable to complete the set with quality repetitions, that means the weight is too great and needs to be readjusted the next time you do these exercises. It is imperative your workouts are always to be done safely and without pain. Also, keep in mind the after effects of the exercise on your mobility and activities of daily living.

You do not need to do strengthening exercises at a maximum effort to effectively gain strength. You will gain strength with sub-maximum effort, which uses the concept of progressive resistance but performed with a lighter resistance that produces a degree of muscle overload, but not at a level of exhaustion.

Remember, the muscle needs to rest to recover from the fatigue, which takes approximately 48 hours. This is why you do not do strength training exercises every day with the same muscle group. You could strengthen the leg muscles one day and the arm muscles the next, but never the same muscle group two days in a row. Please note that as you age it may take longer than 48 hours to recover from your exercise, therefore you may need to adjust your routine to accommodate the changes.

b. Strengthening Equipment

There are different devices and techniques that can help you get stronger, which may include, but are not limited to, the following:

- free weights such as barbells, dumb bells, ankle/wrist weights, and kettle bells.
- resistance machines (they isolate specific muscle groups such as knee flexion, knee extension).
- elastic bands and tubing that provide different resistances, indicated by different colors.
- water exercises using devices such as floatation tubes and dumbbells (push/pull against the resistance of water).
- resistance against your own bodyweight such as push-ups, sit-ups, pull-ups, and slow squats without weights.
- Yoga exercises that use different positions against gravity.
- Pilates, a full body workout that utilizes body positioning and resistance equipment that emphasizes strengthening your core pelvic and shoulder muscles. These exercises are named after Joe Pilates, 1883-1967.
- isometric exercises, which provide resistance when pushing or pulling against an immoveable object.

The type of device or exercise form can also play a role in the strength of your muscles, such as using a free weight to strengthen a specific muscle forces supporting muscles to be exercised more effectively. For example, the biceps is the main muscle (prime mover) used to bend your elbow, along with smaller muscles (accessory muscles: coracobrachialis and brachialis) that steady the motion. This type of strengthening also exercises muscles of the spine, shoulders, and pelvis needed to stabilize the body while the elbow is bending. However, the mechanism of a resistance machine to resist the elbow bending muscles replaces the stabilizing action of the accessory muscles and those of the spine, shoulder and pelvis support muscles, which means these muscles are not exercised as well with machines as with free weights.

c. Developing A Basic Strengthening Routine

There are many types of resistance exercise routines, however to produce the best results follow the basic model of progressive resistance exercises (PRE). The goal of this routine is to find a weight that produces the most resistance by the last set of repetitions. The PRE concept employs two different progressions:

- During one exercise session, increase the resistance with two to three sets of repetitions of one exercise, for example:
  - first set—five pounds ten times
  - second set—ten pounds ten times
  - third set—fifteen pounds ten times.
- Increase the progression of a set of repetitions, for example:
  - for the past three to four exercise sessions, you have been able to successfully accomplish three sets of ten repetitions of five, ten, and fifteen pounds.
  - in the next exercise session add five pounds to each set: do three sets of ten repetitions with ten, fifteen, and twenty pounds, respectively.
  - keep in mind that because of the increased starting weight you may not be able to do all three sets ten times. This is quite normal. You now have a new short-term goal.

◆ each time you reach the goal of doing a progression of resistance and then increase that resistance is a reflection of your strength gain.

d. Variations of the Basic Routine

There are as many strengthening exercise routines as there are philosophies of those who teach them. Consider the following for a maximum benefit of your exercise:

- Do three sets of between eight and twelve repetitions, two to three times a week.

- Consider either of these muscle grouping regimens:

  ◆ do three sets of repetitions for one muscle group before going to the next exercise.

  ◆ do circuit training, which involves repeating a circuit of one set of repetitions for one muscle group, then a different muscle group, and then another, and so on for one cycle. Finally, repeat the same order of exercise with added resistance for a second cycle and then again for the third cycle.

- Alternate the order of the exercises. For example, do an elbow-bending exercise followed by an elbow-straightening exercise. Then do two different exercises that bend and then straighten the joint. There are several advantages to this routine:

  ◆ when you have spasticity of one muscle group, exercising the opposing muscle group helps to calm the spasticity of the first group.

  ◆ exercising one muscle group gives the opposing muscle group a slight chance to rest.

- you can go from one exercise to another with less rest between sets, which improves the efficiency of the exercise routine; it saves time.

- Change the routine when you reach a plateau in your exercise goals. You may have reached your peak of strength or your muscles get bored with this type of routine. In either case, it is beneficial to change the routine by:
  - doing a different number of repetitions and /or sets of the same exercise regimen.
  - changing the order of exercises in that regimen.
  - changing the type of exercise device you are using. For example, if you are using free weights, switch to weight machines for a while.

e. Arm and Leg Strengthening Exercises

Determining exactly which exercises to do is a side trip within your total fitness journey. It is best to first check with your physical therapist as to any muscle strengthening priorities related to your symptoms. Otherwise, have an overall approach to strengthening the main muscle groups that bend and straighten your wrists, elbows, ankles and knee plus the muscles that raise and lower your arms and legs to exercise your shoulders and hips.

f. Core Strengthening Exercises

You may have heard about your core and wondered, *What are they talking about?* Your core mostly refers to all the muscles that attach to your pelvis, spine, and legs. It refers to your abdominal muscles, (of which there are four groups), the buttock muscles, and back muscles. These muscles provide stability for your activities of daily living that involve sitting, standing, bending, twisting, walking, and so on.

The basic concept of the role of strengthening your core is expressed in the axiom, *You cannot shoot a cannon from a canoe.* As your body's movement causes a change in your center of gravity—a point where the average of the weight of different body parts is centered—your core muscles provide postural stability to acclimate to these changes. When these core muscles weaken, those functional activities become more difficult to do. When your core is unstable (like a canoe), the use of your arms and legs (cannons) becomes less effective, challenging your ability to do your activities of daily living, so you become physically unstable.

Strengthening your core muscles involves challenging them with changes of center of gravity from an unstable base. This can be done in a variety of ways, the simplest of which is to sit and move your arms and upper body in different directions with different amounts of weights or resistances. To increase the challenge to these muscles and thus increase their strength, you decrease the stability of the base and increase the amount of change in your center of gravity.

There are many different ways of doing core-strengthening exercises that involve the abdominal muscles, which may include but are not limited to:

- Sitting and balancing on the edge of a chair with good posture, progressing to sitting and balancing on an exercise ball (remember think quality of the exercise).

- Standing with a wide base of support, then progressing to a narrower base and then standing on a spongy pad.

- Bridging exercises that involve lying on your back with your knees bent, upwardly rotating your pelvis thus flatting your back (push your navel toward the floor) and then lifting your buttocks up from the surface, forming a bridge between your feet and your shoulders. From this position your core can be challenged even further by alternately raising and lowering one leg then one arm and then repeating with the other leg and arm. Variations of this exercise may include but are not limited to:

- raising one foot off the surface with the knee bent
- raising one foot off the surface with the knee bent then straightening the knee
- alternating raising and lowering your feet in a marching style
- raising your arms up and then moving them from side to side
- forming a bridge with your shoulders on an exercise ball and feet on the floor then repeating the above exercises.

There are many different ways of doing core-strengthening exercises that involve the buttock and back muscles. If you have a history of back problems or have pain, numbness, or tingling when doing any of the following exercises, consult with a physical therapist before starting or continuing this type of exercise.

The following exercises need to be done on a firm surface while keeping your back and neck in a comfortable position. They may include but are not limited to:

- positioning yourself on your hands and knees, then alternately:
  - raising one arm then the other
  - raising one leg then the other

- - raising one arm and the opposite leg at the same time, then the other pair
- lying facedown (prone) on a firm surface with your arms up next to your head, then alternately:
  - raising one arm then the other
  - raising one leg then the other
  - raising one arm and the opposite leg at the same time, then the other pair
- kneeling with your arms at your side
  - raising one arm then the other
  - raising both arms at the same time
  - holding a weight in each hand then repeating the above exercises

Other exercise regimens that help strengthen your body's core muscles may include, but are not limited to:

- resistance exercises for specific muscles of the abdomen and the back
- rowing exercises
- Pilates
- Yoga
- Tai Chi

Which core strengthening exercise to do is determined by your individual therapeutic needs, but is also determined by safety considerations. For example, if you have difficulty getting down and up off the floor, exercising on a mat might put you at risk of injury after doing the exercise. Instead, consider performing this exercise on a bed or on a raised mat as an alternative. If you have a history of back injury or pain, or you experience back pain while attempting these exercises, stop doing the exercise and consult your healthcare provider.

g. Flexibility Exercises

Flexibility exercises are used to help calm muscle spasticity, help prevent joint and muscle stiffness and delay the onset of muscle soreness (DOMS) after exercise while improving your overall mobility. These exercises include stretching and other activities that promote movement of your joints. Slow stretching allows the muscles to lengthen gradually without triggering spasticity, which would prevent relaxation. The effectiveness of these exercises is based on:

- Stretching slowly—if you stretch too quickly, the muscle may not relax enough, thereby defeating the purpose of the exercise. Furthermore, do not bounce when stretching.

- Moderation—a moderate stretch is somewhere between mild, —which is not enough stretch—and pain—which is too much stretch. Remember that No pain, no gain does not work.

- Time—the length of time for a stretch is dependent on the amount of spasticity and stiffness. The greater the amount of either, the longer you may need to stretch to have the optimal effect while maintaining a moderate stretch. The length of time may vary from several minutes to fifteen to twenty minutes total of doing repetitions of shorter stretching periods. For the length of stretching time, consider each muscle individually; one muscle may need more time than another muscle.

- Frequency—up to a point, the more times you stretch in a day the greater the potential influence on your spasticity. Stretching once a day is generally recommended, but you may need to increase the number of times a day you stretch in order to produce and maintain an optimal effect of the exercise.

A good approach to these exercises is to think of short periods of stretching time with repetitions rather than one long period of stretch without repetition. For example, find a moderate stretch, hold it for ten to fifteen seconds, relieve the stretch for a second or two, and then apply the moderate stretch again for another ten to fifteen seconds. Continue the sequence until you feel relief from the stiffness. Because stretching helps relax a muscle, notice if there is a gain of range of motion increases with each repetition.

Also, note that the best time to strengthen a muscle is right after stretching the opposing muscle. For example, after stretching your calf muscle, practice bending your ankle upward using the muscles on the front part of your lower leg. Alternatively, when you go to strengthen your knee's straightening muscles—the quadriceps, first stretch the knee's bending muscles— the hamstrings. Remember to straighten your knee slowly to help prevent velocity from increasing spasticity of the hamstrings even after they were stretched. Keep in mind that the goal is not to eliminate all spasticity because some of it may help you. You may feel the temporary affects of weakness after stretching, which could interfere with the safe performance of your activities of daily living afterward. This is rare but possible. If it does happen, do not stop doing the exercise, but prepare for its short influence on strength by cutting back on functional activities immediately afterward. This feeling may last several minutes or even longer.

Other exercises to help manage spasticity and stiffness might include gentle Yoga, range of motion, relaxation and meditation, trunk rotation, and alternating movements of your arms and legs. In general, it is best for you to be as active and mobile as safely possible. *Motion is lotion* is a good axiom to use as a reminder of the benefit of movement. Remember, however, to maintain a consistent program of stretching. Consulting with your physical therapist can help you design a program using other exercises that work best for your situation.

h. Endurance Exercises

Endurance exercises help to improve the use of your heart/lung delivery system and the function of your muscles as discussed in a previous chapter. These exercises help to break up the vicious fatigue/rest/more fatigue cycle, however there are other possible benefits that may include, but are not limited to:

- decreasing fatigue
- increasing strength
- improving spasticity and bladder management
- improving ability to complete activities of daily living
- increasing sense of quality of life
- reduce the risk factors of cardiovascular and lung diseases.

The heart of this process involves becoming fatigued in a healthy way through appropriate exercise. It may sound conflicting that you have to become fatigued to manage your energy; however, endurance exercise is a way to break up this vicious cycle. It also involves utilizing energy-management skills and the concept that you cannot speed up the process, which means it may take some time before you begin to feel the benefits. Utilizing the concept of delayed gratification learned through your emotional health and cognitive well-being concepts will help you maintain the discipline to stick to the program. Again, always check with your health care provider before starting any new exercise routine.

1. Cardiopulmonary Endurance Exercises

Cardio or aerobic exercises are based on the gradual progression of increased heart rate, exertion of breathing, frequency, and time. When you increase the demand on your muscles, whether through exercise or functional activities such as walking up a flight of stairs, your heart rate and breathing rate will normally go up. This is a response to the increased call for the cardiopulmonary transportation cycle to deliver more oxygen and nutrients to your cells and the removal of carbon dioxide and other waste products from your cells. To improve your overall endurance, you need to gradually increase that demand on your muscles, heart, and lungs through an appropriate increase of effort over time.

A measurement of this demand on your heart and lungs can be determined by taking your pulse during your exercise. There are several ways to take your pulse:

- Place your first and second fingers on your carotid artery, which is found in the groove of the strap muscle in your neck or place the fingers on the palm side of your wrist at the base of your thumb; do not press too hard.
- Count the number of heartbeats for ten seconds and multiply by six to find the number of beats per minute.
- Wear a heart rate monitor

Your goal in this type of endurance exercise is to reach a target heart rate. A simple, though somewhat inaccurate method of measuring this point of exertion is to exercise at approximately eighty percent of the sum of two hundred twenty minus your age. For example, if you were forty years old, your target heart rate would be approximately one hundred forty four beats per minute [.80 x (220-40) = .80 times (180) = 144]. However, the best way to determine your individual target heart rate is to have a metabolic test that may be obtained through your health care provider or at a local health club.

Another measurement of this demand on your heart and lungs can be determined by monitoring your breathing rate, which is measured through your perceived exertion. What this means is that as your heart rate goes up, so does your breathing rate. When you reach your target heart rate as described above, your breathing rate will be somewhat labored. Ideally, you need to be at an exercise intensity to produce a breathing rate and depth that would prevent you from finishing a normal sentence without having to take a breath; this is your target perceived exertion. On a scale of zero to ten (modified Borg scale), where zero is no effort and ten is maximum effort, a therapeutic perceived exertion would be around four or five.

Gradually increase your heart rate and perceived exertion to target levels over time by increasing the intensity of the exercise, specifically increasing the minutes per session and number of times a week you exercise. You cannot rush the process, which means that going beyond your target heart rate and perceived exertion does not speed up or increase the results of the exercise and may even hinder the process. Stick to the guidelines to provide an optimum response to your efforts.

The use of target heart rate and perceived exertion as a means of measuring optimum training levels is very subjective and variable from person to person. They can be influenced by your MS symptoms, prescription medications you may be taking, and the possibility that you may be part of a small numbers of people with MS whose heart and breathing rates do not go up in accordance with demand. Check with your health care provider if you suspect you fit into any of these possibilities.

There are different exercises you can use to increase endurance, which include, but are not limited to, the following:

- outdoor bicycling or stationary bicycling
- running outdoors or on a treadmill
- swimming
- stair master
- rowing machine
- upper-body cycling

2. Muscular Endurance Exercises

You could increase muscle endurance by repeating a low-resistance strengthening exercise with higher repetitions. For example, instead of doing three sets of eight to twelve repetitions of a maximum resistance as with strengthening exercises, lower the resistance and do three sets of twenty repetitions. This type of exercise program is best discussed with your physical therapist about what is best for your situation.

i. Other Exercises

There are other physical therapy-oriented types of exercises that address specific MS symptoms that could be incorporated into your self-management program. These exercises are best determined by your physical therapist, which may include but are not limited to:

- Balance—Many balance exercises incorporate core-strengthening exercises along with ways of stimulating the brain's balance centers. The exercises might include standing on uneven surfaces, sitting with different levels of stability, and changes of weight from one side to another while sitting or standing.

- Coordination—There are exercises that challenge your arm and leg muscles in slower controlled movements to help improve hand-eye coordination. These may include exercises for the smaller muscles of hand and larger movements of the arms and legs.

- Pelvic floor—Kegel exercises will help strengthen the muscles that line the floor of your pelvis that can be used in bladder management.

INTEGRATING SYMPTOM MANAGEMENT WITH PHYSICAL FITNESS

A wise man should consider that health is the greatest of human blessings, and learn how by his own thought to derive benefit from his illnesses.

Hippocrates (460–370 BC;
ancient Greek physician)

Symptom Management

There is growing scientific, medical research that supports the concepts of fitness as having a direct and indirect effect on managing the symptoms of multiple sclerosis. Ultimately, the goal of living well with MS is self-management. This concept is supported through your emotional health and cognitive well-being because it requires relationships with your care-partners, who may have to provide a direct role in your symptom management, and with your team of health care providers who may prescribe medications, treatments, and equipment. The overall goal of self-management is to improve your function, maintain safety, and prevent complications directly through your intervention, which are the same ambitions and end results of living well with MS.

There are some symptoms, such as fatigue and spasticity, that daily management is necessary and on which fitness can have a positive influence. However, the possible daily fluctuations of these symptoms and others may impact your fitness goals. Dealing with this situation can be emotionally taxing and at times overwhelming, but with the teamwork of all involved you can be successful.

An important element in these self-management efforts is paying close attention to how the daily variables of your symptoms affect your activities and how your activities affect your symptoms. Learning the causes and effects for each symptom individually and their interactions with other symptoms collectively may help you weather these day-to-day fluctuations. Keep in mind there are variables over which you have no control. For example, hot environments will increase fatigue. With this knowledge, you can avoid becoming overheated, yet you can still become fatigued because of some other variable of fatigue not in your control. Even though fatigue seems unavoidable, being knowledgeable of other possible variables will help you overcome the frustration of seemingly being out of control of the situation. Learning how to adapt your energy expenditure may have at least some influence over the negative outcome for this period of time being influenced by effects beside heat-related fatigue.

There are many tips that can help with your daily responsibilities of symptom management. Some you may discover on your own through trial and error, some you learn from others with MS, and some you learn from your health care providers. It is most important to find what works and does not work for your situation. Always keep in mind they should not conflict with your health care providers' recommendations. For example, always check with your providers before taking herbal and vitamin supplements, as they may be incompatible with your medications or too much of one could be toxic.

a. Muscle Weakness

There are three ways in which your muscles may lose strength, two of which are not reversible and one that has the potential for reversal:

- the MS disease process—this is not reversible at this time
- aging—is also nonreversible
- inactivity—potentially reversible.

However, no matter the cause, when muscles weaken they get smaller and less efficient; they go through atrophy. Only muscle loss not directly affected by your MS and aging are reversible through exercise, but sometimes it is difficult to tell which is which. It is very important to remember that inactivity causes weakness and atrophy. It may be impossible to determine whether muscle weakness is due to reversible or non-reversible causes unless you begin an exercise program and see whether muscle strength and condition are improved. Your health care provider may be able to help you determine that difference. No matter the cause, exercise will help to either strengthen the reversible or maintain what is left after the non-reversible causes have done their damage.

b. Spasticity

Spasticity is caused by your multiple sclerosis affecting the nerves that normally allow relaxation of your muscles. This results in a conflict between the muscles that straighten your joints and those that bend them. Spasticity can be described as the body's compensation for weakness, which means there can be good spasticity that helps maintain function as opposed to bad spasticity that interferes with function.

Spasticity is velocity or speed-related, which means the lack of relaxation increases the faster you stretch the muscle. For example, in the motion of your knee, if the hamstring muscles that bend the knee have spasticity and do not relax quickly enough, they will work against the quadriceps muscles that are trying to straighten the knee. The faster the motion, the less relaxation of the opposing muscles. This causes a reduction of the smoothness of motion, such as with walking. For example, if the motion of walking is sped up to result in running, the spastic hamstring muscles will further resist knee-straightening, resulting in a more noticeable effect on function. This conflict with spasticity between the muscle groups results in an increase in work of the muscles and contributes to more fatigue.

Spasticity may interfere with your ability to move fluidly and carry out your activities of daily living efficiently and safely. If mild enough, it may be managed with exercise. Moderate spasticity is usually managed with exercise and medications, the latter of which in high doses tend to cause grogginess and even weakness. Severe spasticity may be managed with a pump (Intrathecal Baclofen Pump), which is surgically placed under the skin of the abdomen and pumps a liquid medication through a small tube into your spinal cord to bathe the nerves that go to the affected muscles. This allows precise amounts of medication needed to help manage the spasticity without the groggy affects of the oral medications, which are eliminated. Botox® injections and some other surgical procedures have also been used to help manage severely debilitating spasticity. Always consult your health care provider as to appropriate spasticity management for your situation.

Be aware that pain, infection, dehydration, and other irritations may exaggerate spasticity. For example, bladder irritation along with lack of appropriate fluid intake when you restrict fluids because of urinary frequency and urgency may increase spasticity of the legs. Tell your health care provider of any abnormal increases in your spasticity, which may be a sign of fever and pain due to infection. When the irritations are reduced or removed spasticity will most likely return to its own level. This exaggerated spasticity is often referred to as a pseudo-exacerbation or false flare up.

c. Stiffness

Prolonged inactivity causes your muscles, tendons, and joint tissues to become stiff and difficult to move. This results in fatigue and interference with efficient and safe activities of daily living. Over long periods of being immobile, these tissues may become permanently stiff. One adage to remember about spasticity and stiffness is *Motion is lotion*. Movement, whether through stretching exercises or activities of daily living, can be a lubricant for your muscles and joints.

d. Balance

Balance difficulties may be a result of any combination of other possible influences caused by your multiple sclerosis, which may affect:

- Parts of the brain that control balance (vestibular system of the inner ear).
- Loss of sensation in the feet. If you cannot feel your feet it is difficult for the brain to provide feedback to the rest of the body to maintain balance.
- Loss of your brain's sense of body position in space (proprioception), such as not knowing exactly where your foot is when you cannot see it.
- Uneven muscle strength resulting in one leg being stronger than the other.
- Poor control of your pelvis because of weak core muscles, which connect your legs and spine to your pelvis.

- Spasticity of leg muscles, especially if there is more spasticity in one leg than another.

- Low vision and other vision difficulties, which can impact how you are able to use visual cues to tell your body how to move in space.

Loss of balance may also have a great influence on your mobility, which may cause you to:

- Fall and injure yourself.

- Walk with a stagger (ataxia), which may cause you to fatigue sooner and may be perceived by others as you being under the influence of alcohol or drugs.

- Use more physical energy to maintain your upright posture and to prevent yourself from falling, which may cause you to fatigue sooner.

As a result of your loss of balance you may find yourself engaging in insecure wall walking or furniture walking, which may cause you to misjudge the distance and stability of the object for which you are reaching. In the presence of fatigue, this could cause you to fall and injure yourself. If you find yourself using these or other risky ways of modifying your mobility to accommodate to balance problems, it would be beneficial to use one or more adaptive aids to maintain your safety (see the list in the section Mobility).

f. Mobility

Your ability to perform activities of daily living and get from one point to another is very important to your overall quality of life. There are factors related to your multiple sclerosis that may influence your ability to maintain your mobility, which may include, but are not limited to:

- fatigue

- spasticity and stiffness
- leg muscle weakness
- uneven muscle strength
- visual disturbances
- balance problems.

There are different mobility devices that are available to help you accommodate to the factors that limit your mobility. It is best to check with your physical therapist to identify which mobility device and training is appropriate for your circumstance. Some of these aids were listed under energy management, but as a reminder, the following my be considered to help you complete tasks more effectively, efficiently, and safely.

- Use canes, crutches, and walkers for balance and weakness problems.
- Wear splints and braces for weakness and paralysis.
- Use a walker with a seat to sit on when you get tired and a basket in which to carry objects.
- Use a wheelchair for long distances; many stores and malls have both electrically powered or manual wheelchairs available for your use. Airports have customer service representatives who will transport you to your destination within the airport.
- Use brighter lighting and contrast of colors and brightness to help differentiate changes in levels or surfaces, such as going from tile or hardwood flooring to carpeting.
- Be aware of different levels of surfaces, such as with doorsills and steps.
- Remove throw rugs and other objects that shift or move with contact.

- Use bathroom safety equipment, such as a shower chair or tub transfer bench and handheld showers.

- Rearrange furniture to allow for a wider path of travel.

- Obtain a handicapped parking permit through your state licensing bureau.

Aids are important tools to help you live your life safely and with dignity. However, you may be reluctant to use any of them for one of several reasons:

- You may feel you are giving into the disease.

- You may feel that other people will think you are lazy or taking the easy way out of doing something.

- You may think of yourself as being more efficient and therefore able to do more.

- You might have a fear of being labeled disabled, which may be a self-imposed label developed through negative experiences with other people with disabilities.

It may take some time to work through these perceptions, but remember they are self-imposed. Not everyone will perceive you in negative ways and, for those who are bothered by it, let it be their problem. When you acclimate to the disease, it is as if you were reacting to a change in weather, which you have no control over other than to change your clothes.

You may think that once you use an aid you will always have to use it. One way to tackle this matter is to realize that you use what you need to be functional with that particular situation. It is similar to wearing sunglasses when it is sunny and reading glasses when you need to read. You use the device that adapts to your situation. For example, you can normally handle walking short distances without a lot of difficulty, though you may feel somewhat fatigued afterward.

However, if you need to walk long distances, such as when shopping at the local mall, it could be very difficult to complete without putting yourself at risk of falling because of severe fatigue. In that situation, using a wheelchair would be a prudent choice. Many malls and large stores have power wheelchairs you can borrow for the shopping duration. Again, use the device that best suits your situation at the time.

The most important concepts of mobility management are safety and energy efficiency. Do what you need to do to maintain those concepts despite how others may perceive you. While there are many self-defeating attitudes that may hold you back from being functional and independent, a lot of your reluctance is based on your perception of your self and your sensitivity to other's perceptions of you. Use the concepts of emotional health and cognitive well-being to help you address these issues.

Bladder Dysfunction

You may not have thought of your urinary system and bladder management as being a part of your physical fitness, but they do play a very important role in keeping your body healthy. MS may affect this essential bodily function and your fitness may help manage it.

a. Urinary System Function

The urinary tract is made up of the following:

- Two kidneys—found close to your spine and under the last two ribs of the chest wall
- Ureters—tubes that go from your kidneys to your bladder

- The bladder—a muscular sac (detrusor) that stores and eliminates urine
- Sphincters—valves that help control bladder emptying
- Urethra—a tube that goes from the bladder to outside of the body.

The kidneys filter your blood of metabolic waste by-products, help to maintain a balance of a variety of electrolytes (dissolved salts), help maintain the body's fluid balance, and produce urine. The amount of urine produced varies depending on physical activity, consumption of fluids, and ingestion of foods containing various salts.

The bladder and the urethra use the opening and closing of the sphincters (valves) to allow filling and emptying. Normally, the bladder fills at a fairly consistent rate (approximately two ounces or sixty milliliters an hour) and when it reaches a certain volume (approximately twelve ounces or three hundred sixty milliliters) you feel the need to empty your bladder. You are normally able to resist this urge for a while by using the muscles of your pelvic floor to act like a scissor valve to prevent emptying, but the bladder continues to fill until you reach a point where you have to give in and get to a bathroom. To empty your bladder, the pelvic floor muscles relax, the valves open, the bladder squeezes, and you void your bladder of urine, leaving very little urine left afterward. The normal amount of this residual urine is normally less than approximately three and one half ounces (100 milliliters), however if it is repeatedly greater than this amount, there is an increased risk of bladder infection.

Multiple sclerosis can affect normal bladder function, producing several of the possible situations:

- Your pelvic floor muscles may have weakened and are unable to squeeze strongly enough to hold back the urge to empty your bladder.

- You could have a limp or flaccid bladder that does not create enough pressure to completely empty. This is not uncommon in women who have gone through childbirth.

- You could have a tight or spastic bladder where the need to go is triggered at a lower volume of urine, forcing you to empty your bladder more often. If this pressure gets too high, it could force urine back up toward the kidneys, which could cause infection, permanent damage, and could possibly be life threatening.

- You could have poor coordination between your bladder muscle and the valves that open and close to control urine flow. The bladder tries to empty, but the valves do not open or the valves open when you do not want the bladder to empty.

These bladder conditions may result in urgency, frequency, and incontinence that are frustrating and embarrassing and may lead to social isolation. The exact cause of these symptoms and the best management techniques can only be assessed through thorough urological exams. If you have any of these symptoms, consult with your health care provider.

b. Hydration

Maintaining appropriate levels of fluid intake or hydration is very important in various bodily functions, especially muscular activity. Yet, you may have a tendency to neglect this vital concept because of increased urgency and frequency of urination associated with your multiple sclerosis. There are possible consequences of not drinking enough fluids, which may include, but are not limited to increases in:

- fatigue
- spasticity
- muscle weakness
- bladder infections
- controlling body temperature.

The balance and timing of hydration play an important role in the health of your urinary system, the management of which involves appropriate bladder maintenance.

c. Bladder Management

A healthy urinary tract relies on coordinated efforts between you and your health care provider to provide good fluid management, adequate bladder emptying, and appropriate exercise. However, there are some useful self-managing tips that may add to, but do not replace, the treatment prescribed by your health care provider. For fluid intake:

- try to maintain an even intake of fluids throughout the day, totaling approximately sixty-four ounces (eighteen hundred milliliters).
- try to drink approximately sixteen ounces (four hundred milliliters) at meals and approximately eight ounces (two hundred milliliters) between meals, basically two hours apart.
- if you restrict fluids too much to avoid urinating too many times, you may become dehydrated. Dehydration can cause fatigue, increased spasticity, and increased risk of bladder infection.

- keep in mind that ice cream, gelatin products, puddings, yogurt, soups, and other creamy type products contribute to your total fluid intake.

- stop taking in fluids approximately four hours before bedtime to help reduce nighttime frequency.

- avoid beverages that contain caffeine, citrus, and carbonation, as they tend to irritate the bladder.

- avoid alcohol because it stimulates more urine production.

Salty foods in large amounts may cause retention of fluids resulting in puffiness, especially of the feet and lower legs; however, this fluid may be released when you lie down, causing an increase in urine production.

Try to empty your bladder at regular intervals of approximately every three and a half to four hours throughout the day. Take your time in urinating. Your bladder can rush you, but you cannot rush it.

Never try to force urine out of your bladder by pushing hard on the lower part of your abdomen or by straining to empty, unless you are instructed to do so by your health care provider.

To help completely empty your bladder, try any or all of the following techniques:

- sit down to urinate. Yes, men that means you too. Women, this means no hovering.

- lean forward with your forearms on your thighs, relax and allow the bladder to empty. Remember, no straining unless instructed to so by your health care provider.

- try to stimulate urination by creating a gentle pressure using your fingers over your lower abdomen to find a spot that stimulates the feeling of wanting to urinate. This sweet spot might be found in more than one area.

- if you find a sweet spot, place the tips of your first and second fingers over the area, then gently push and release rapidly for three or four beats, relax and wait five or six seconds. If nothing happens, try again. If urine does start to flow, relax and let your bladder empty some more and remember not to strain.

- repeat as often as you are successful.

- if you are not successful after three or four attempts, stop trying and try a different sweet spot if you can find another.

- try wiping the end of your urethra with a piece of toilet paper, then relax and wait five or six seconds. If nothing happens, try another technique.

- try standing up and waiting five or six seconds. If you feel a slight urge, sit down and try to relax and void some more.

- try the following breathing exercises:
  - lean forward with your forearms on your thighs and relax
  - exhale a moderate amount of air from your lungs, then hold your breath
  - draw in your abdomen as deep as possible without inhaling and then breathe in as you let your abdomen balloon outward.

If the treatment program and self-management techniques are not effective in reducing or coping with the symptoms, your health care provider may prescribe intermittent bladder catheterization, which involves placing a sterile catheter in your bladder that empties into a toilet. You may be instructed to perform this technique every three to four hours or when urgency arises. This is generally not a difficult procedure, and you may be able to do it independently with a little practice unless you have tremors, weakness, or paralysis of your hands . Cleanliness is very important to help prevent urinary tract infections. Your health care provider will instruct you how to perform the procedure appropriately and indicate the signs and symptoms of infection.

If you are unable to use an intermittent catheter independently because of hand coordination, have difficulty getting on and off the toilet efficiently and safely, or if you are having frequent incontinence and infection, an indwelling catheter could be used. This type of catheter is inserted into the bladder and sealed with an inflatable balloon to prevent leaks. The catheter is attached to a collection bag that can be emptied periodically. The indwelling catheter needs to be changed on occasion and appropriate amounts of liquid need to be consumed to maintain a healthy urinary system. Your health care provider will help you manage these situations. However, no matter the method of bladder management a healthy urologic system is of utmost importance.

Kegel exercises can be incorporated into your bladder management scheme to help strengthen the muscles that line the floor of your pelvis and help stave off sudden urges of urination by squeezing the urethra as this tube passes through these pelvic floor muscles. Aerobic and pelvic core strengthening exercises have been cited as helping contribute to bladder management. Consult with your physical therapist to learn how to do these exercises appropriately.

STAYING ON A LIVING WELL JOURNEY

One of the goals of physical fitness is to help manage the symptoms of your multiple sclerosis. Integrating this goal into your lifestyle requires the other two components of living well with MS: admitting that you have no control over your MS while having the desire to influence your response to multiple sclerosis over which do you have some control. That is the essence of emotional health and to know the difference between two by having an understanding of MS and physical fitness concepts is the basis of cognitive well-being.

Starting and sticking to an exercise program whether for general fitness or symptoms management can very difficult. It takes time, energy, and persistence to maintain a routine of exercises that is beneficial; however, the rewards of your efforts will far outweigh any inconveniences. Tips to maintain an exercise program may include, but are not limited to thefollowing ideas:

- Do a little bit frequently during the day (three to five minutes at a time, several times a day) This is less overwhelming than doing a thirty- or sixty-minute program.

- Use photos or visual reminders of your exercises to assist you to remember to do them.

- Link your exercises to other daily tasks- for example: do your ankle stretch after you get a drink of water, or do a slow sit to stand exercise during TV show changes.

- Write down and track your participation; make a check mark next to each exercise after it is completed.

- Reward yourself: If you have reached your goal for the week, reward yourself with a positive reinforcement such as spending more time your family, going to a movie, having occasional ice cream cone, and so on.

As you experience breakdowns and breakthroughs, learn from the experiences and channel what you learn about yourself into positive outcomes for you and others.

EPILOGUE

Desire is the starting point of all achievement, not a hope, not a wish, but a keen pulsating desire which transcends everything.

– **Napoleon Hill** (1883–1970; American writer)

Living with the progressive nature of multiple sclerosis can be a difficult, challenging journey complicated by an array of detours and roadblocks. The skills and knowledge gained through the concepts of living well with MS can help you successfully navigate present and future barriers. Medical research continues to support the concepts of living well as a means of positively managing many of the complexities of MS. While multiple sclerosis and living well may seem incompatible to you, it is the very reason they must co-exist. Multiple sclerosis breaks down, whereas living well builds up. However, living well is not a single entity, but composed of three domains: emotional health, cognitive well-being, and physical fitness.

Emotional Health

Emotional health involves the process of redefining your self in positive ways despite the negative circumstances of having multiple sclerosis. Like all aspects of fitness, emotional fitness needs to be reinforced constantly and positively. While living with multiple sclerosis is complex and variable, your reaction to your MS can be positive. As you experience the fluctuations of life in general, understanding the various levels and each concept within your emotional health on which you could travel may help you contend with these changes more positively. Reaching a personality because of your reaction to your multiple sclerosis does not mean you will remain there. You may revert to a less productive personality as your MS progresses or when you have change in other aspects of your life. You need to work continuously at moving upward in levels, even when you have a negative breakdown along your journey. When these occur, you need to look for positive breakthroughs to bring you back on the road toward a higher-functioning personality.

In addition to working continuously at achieving higher levels of an emotional personality, attending self-help groups led by a trained facilitator may help you deal with this roller-coaster ride. However, serious emotional upheaval needs to be addressed by a mental health care provider who is professionally trained to treat these situations.

Another source of support is your spirituality. Having an emotional healthy spirituality will help you through all transitions in life, but particularly when you are confronted with adversity. Seeking out support from your clergy may be as important as seeking out support from a mental health care provider.

The concepts of emotional health are vital in obtaining optimum wellness and are based on the following key points:

- Break out of your emotional shell. Living in a cocoon composed of the instant gratification of food and negative reinforcement of rest to avoid fatigue leads to the complications of poor nutrition and inactivity. To improve your emotional fitness you need to remove the misleading protective defenses of apathy, victimization, and survival.

- Stop living in your story. Get out of the ground-hog-day scenario of living in the accounts regarding your losses and begin to find the good in your situation.

- Take ownership of your MS. Just like owning a car or home, it is your MS and you are responsible for its care and management.

- Let go of the past. The past is over; it is behind you. Creating possibilities for the future and acting upon them in the present will produce change.

- Never give up hope. Hope is a part of your future thinking of living a life without multiple sclerosis.

- Begin to build on your successes. In the midst of all the negativity of MS lay the seeds of success; water them and let them grow.

- Find strength in your weakness through faith. You are not alone in your grief and loss; find strength in a power beyond your humanism.

- Seek ways to redefine your self positively. The self that lies within you goes beyond the negativity of having MS; find the positive in your views of who you are.

- If you are not creating change, it is creating you. Change is always occurring whether you like it or not; be the change you wish to see.

- Turn negative circumstances into positive outcomes. There is good in your life with MS, however you need to search for it and channel it to help others and, in turn, help yourself.

- Get out of the bleachers. Sitting in the bleachers of hope as a cheerleader does not directly contribute to the outcome of the game. Get on to the playing field of volunteering and fundraising to be an active part of your destiny of living without MS.

Wellness cannot be built on a foundation of the shifting sands of being a victim or survivor. It needs to be built upon the solid rock of being proactive and an advocate that are fed and nurtured through the concepts of mental and physical fitness.

Cognitive Well-Being

Cognitive well-being involves learning and relearning over time. The more you know about your MS and your overall health, the better you are able to know how they affect you and how you can manage them. These concepts will help you have a better understanding of your situation, which will help you prepare for a future that is unknown. There are many learning opportunities for you to explore. Take advantage of them and keep your mind as sharp as possible. Your health care provider and the National MS Society are available to help you with these endeavors. All these factors will help you with your total well-being, reinforce your emotional health, and help you understand the need for physical fitness.

Cognitive well-being can be obtained through the following concepts:

- Improve your total health literacy. Become knowledgeable of all aspects of your health, for MS may not be your only health concern.

- Become an expert in your multiple sclerosis. Knowing as much about your MS as possible increases your ability to help manage it.

- Be proactive in your total health care. Multiple sclerosis is not the only disease you may encounter.

Contact a primary care physician to use the principles of preventive medicine in avoiding heart disease, diabetes, cancers, and other possible diseases. Do not smoke, follow recommended dietary strategies, exercise, and follow disease-screening guidelines.

- Prepare now for your future with MS. Multiple sclerosis is a progressive disease. Preparing now will lessen the impact for possible changes in employment, finances, medical insurance, housing, and accessibility.

- Exercise your brain. Your brain needs a workout as well as your body to stay in shape. Read, play word and board games, and do crossword puzzles and other mental exercises.

- Optimize your cognitive function. Explore ways of adapting to any cognitive problems you may be experiencing with attention, memory, or executive function

Physical Fitness

Physical fitness is the driving force of total fitness while also maintaining the assistance of the emotional health and cognitive well-being concepts. Physical fitness is an important component of self-management that can be integrated into your MS symptom management program by looking at efficient ways to perform exercises that are developed by your physical therapist and ones you may add on your own. Physical fitness is deemed safe and effective by medical research. It needs to be included in the overall management of your multiple sclerosis. The concepts of physical fitness consist of the following:

- What you do not use, you lose. You lose strength and endurance if you use your muscles just for activities of daily living. You need to exercise to fill the gap created by what you used to be able to do and what you can do now.

- You cannot do it alone. Seek help through your health care provider, local fitness resources, and the National MS Society to help you find the best setting to get started.

- Start slowly and consider the aftereffects. You want your body to react positively to exercise. If you try to do too much too soon, you may cause pain and increased fatigue, which may discourage you from exercising.

- Be persistent, for it is not the day it is the habit. Doing something to add to your physical fitness will benefit you even if is not like the day before.

- Be patient. It takes weeks, months, and even years to feel the full benefit of physical fitness. Think of the story of the tortoise and the hare.

- Rely on positive reinforcement and delayed gratification. The results of your efforts to increase strength, flexibility, and endurance take time. Observe your gradual improvement in function to help strengthen your resolve to become physically fit.

- Prepare for a future of being free from the physical confines of multiple sclerosis. Physical fitness helps undo the negative affects of inactivity, but not the direct affects of MS. However, becoming physically fit now will better prepare you for the rigors of the rehabilitation during which you will need to exercise to restore your body when the cure and reversal of multiple sclerosis is available.

- Follow a nutritionally sound diet. To fuel an exercising body and help keep an appropriate body weight requires proper nutrition.

- Follow healthy lifestyle choices. If you smoke or consume excess amounts of alcohol, stop.

Physical fitness feeds the advocate in you. The concepts of emotional health are supported through your physical fitness efforts. As your fitness grows, you are better able to adapt to the emotional challenges of MS.

Integrating Symptom Management with Fitness

Self-management is a basic part of the overall management of your multiple sclerosis and is directly related to your total fitness:

- Emotional health—taking responsibility
- Cognitive well-being—being an expert in your MS
- Physical fitness—exercising and managing symptoms

An important concept of self-management is one of energy management, which requires an awareness of how fatigue—the common MS symptom—affects your activities of daily living. In summary it involves the following:

- pacing your total day and individual activities with intermittent activity and rest
- avoiding increases of your core body temperature

- exercising to improve overall fitness
- maintaining an appropriate body weight
- managing your spasticity
- following a bladder-management program
- maintaining a healthy well-rounded diet
- getting adequate sleep
- using adaptive equipment for stability and long distances when needed
- consulting with a mental-health professional for depression
- consulting with your health care provider for possible use of medical treatment for other causes of low energy.

Incorporating the concepts of managing symptoms through fitness cannot be done alone. To avoid complications of any misdirected management tool, it is best to coordinate your total management with your health care providers. This is especially important when it comes to symptom management and exercises as a part of that management.

Staying on a Living Well Journey

Maintaining a living well journey takes time, dedication, discipline and due diligence toward your mission. Because of life's various stressors and circumstances, plus having multiple sclerosis, you are confronted with breakdowns in your journey. Some of them may be monumental. Relying upon the principles of emotional health will help you overcome these detours to the best of your ability. It is imperative to try to do something during these hard times, depending on the circumstances. If you have a major exacerbation of your MS, you will need to follow the recommendations of your health care providers. If you experience a less traumatic life-altering event, try finding a balance between dealing with it and your living well program.

You can think of the various speed bumps of life as opportunities to learn, to grow, and to accommodate to their demands. Each is a fork in the road that forces you to make a decision about which way to go. The strength and resolve you gain through your living well journey can help you smooth the road and create healthy directions toward your destiny: to be free from the confines of multiple sclerosis.

Accept the challenge of living well with multiple sclerosis and have a great journey!

> *The most glorious moments in your life are not the so-called days of success, but rather those days when out of dejection and despair you feel rise in you a challenge to life, and the promise of future accomplishments.*
>
> *—**Gustavo Flaubert** (1821–1880; French novelist)*